ADHD

The Ultimate ADHD Handbook and Guide For Parents

(Survival Guide to Help Teens Improve Their Motivation and Confidence)

Otto Livingston

MW00508863

Published By Jordan Levy

Otto Livingston

All Rights Reserved

ADHD: The Ultimate ADHD Handbook and Guide For Parents (Survival Guide to Help Teens Improve Their Motivation and Confidence)

ISBN 978-1-77485-292-7

All rights reserved. No part of this guide may be reproduced in any form without permission in writing from the publisher except in the case of brief quotations embodied in critical articles or reviews.

Legal & Disclaimer

The information contained in this book is not designed to replace or take the place of any form of medicine or professional medical advice. The information in this book has been provided for educational and entertainment purposes only.

The information contained in this book has been compiled from sources deemed reliable, and it is accurate to the best of the Author's knowledge; however, the Author cannot guarantee its accuracy and validity and cannot be held liable for any errors or omissions. Changes are periodically made to this book. You must consult your doctor or get professional medical advice before using any of the suggested remedies, techniques, or information in this book.

Upon using the information contained in this book, you agree to hold harmless the Author from and against any damages, costs, and expenses, including any legal fees potentially resulting from the application of any of the information provided by this guide. This disclaimer applies to any damages or injury caused by the use and application, whether directly or indirectly, of any advice or information presented, whether for breach of contract, tort, negligence, personal injury, criminal intent, or under any other cause of action.

You agree to accept all risks of using the information presented inside this book. You need to consult a professional medical practitioner in order to ensure you are both able and healthy enough to participate in this program.

Table of Contents

Introduction

ADD also known as ADHD has always been an unfavourable connotation for a lot of people. People with this disorder are not good in any way and are merely being a burden for their families and communities. Perhaps because of their inability of concentration on the task at hand, their inability to settle, and the chaos that they create in the classrooms , as well as at home.

Although the attention deficit hyperactivity disorder appears to alter what is as normal or typical, this disorder can be controlled and managed when it is not overgrown. Actually, ADHD is not all about negatives if we look at how it has changed the lives of a lot of famous individuals. The comedian Jim Carrey, for instance has had to cope with his ADHD through being the class clown. He didn't realize that his condition could one day lead him to Hollywood. Diagnosed with ADHD in the college years, Extreme Makeover: Home Edition host Ty Pennington had lots of energy and determination to conquer, so carpentry became a way to express. Soon the builder was building homes for other people through his reality show, which is telecast around the world.

In the case of Olympian Michael Phelps, swimming was his method of dealing to his ADHD and later went through the process of winning 14 gold medals in the Athens and Beijing Olympics. It's been said that Hollywood's Will Smith had trouble paying attention at a young age but it didn't hinder him from becoming a popular actor and singer who today. In the same way, ADD did not prevent the Grammy-award-winning musician Justin Timberlake from making a name for himself in the world of showbiz.

Virgin Sir Richard Branson, the founder of Virgin Airlines,'s anxiety due to ADHD was later the reason he decided to start an airline that was a major one. Branson was also a dreamer of taking visitors into space, and even imagined an underwater aircraft and a spaceship, which eventually was realized. Similar to that, JetBlue founder David Neeleman was successful because of and despite having ADHD. In reality, Neeleman credits his ADHD for his success, saying "with ADHD comes innovation as well as the capacity to see out of boundaries."

Jamie Oliver had to resort to healthy eating , which helped him control his illness and eventually turn him into the world's most famous chef. James Carville, a political expert and commentator has been credited with directing campaign for the the former US Secretary of State Bill Clinton and former British Prime Minister Tony Blair.

From being an "troublemaker" at the school environment, Pete Rose became a Major League Baseball star while Terry Bradshaw, the former NFL quarterback who won his Pittsburgh Steelers four

Super Bowl titles, was plagued by ADHD when he was a kid.

Socialite and hotel heiress Paris Hilton also has ADHD as does Deal or No Deal host Howie Mandel.

The most important thing to remember is: ADD/ADHD might cause problems for the sufferer and their family members However, it isn't a problem that is out of manageable. For many sufferers, the condition has been a path toward success.

Are yourself or your kid been diagnosed with ADHD or ADD? Don't be depressed. Consider what these amazing people have achieved in spite of having ADHD or ADD. You too can overcome this condition and lead a fulfilling and fulfilling life. It is possible to consider that having ADHD is a blessing disguise.

Chapter 1: What is Adhd?

ADHD Preview

He was always an annoyance from the moment he was able to be able to move. Even as a child when he was a toddler, he would rip through the house, leaving an unintentional trail screaming at the high pitch as he climbed over and down furniture and other items. This is the son of Prima, Jeremiah. There was nothing that would keep his attention for more than a few minutes and, in most cases, he'd leave without warning and showed little awareness of the dangers of crowds in malls and bustling streets.

Prima was able to see the exhausting parenting routine during the first few years, based on the idea that Boys are boys. But at the point that Jeremiah was eight years old and still not slowing down. He was getting more difficult to manage. It was difficult to make him get his attention to even the most basic of tasks, including chores and homework.

Then the comments of his teachers regarding him being unobservant and disruptive during class started pouring into. The comments seemed okay initially, but the frequency increased and Prima was unable to ignore them any further. Prima took him to a doctor and the doctor recommended that he undergo an assessment for attention deficit disorder (ADHD) assessment.

ADHD affects approximately 10% of school-age children, making it a very common behavioral disorder. While no one is sure why it isn't yet understood, ADHD is 3 times more common among males than females.

Children who suffer from ADHD are extremely active, move without thinking and are having issues with concentration. While they can comprehend what they need to do when being told however, they struggle with doing what they've been instructed to do since they can't remain in one spot for long, pay attention to particulars or pay attention.

It is not uncommon for children, particularly the younger ones, to exhibit this behavior certain times, particularly when they're excited or nervous, children suffering from ADHD suffer from these signs throughout their lives for a lengthy time, and can be seen in a variety of situations. The symptoms can hinder how the child performs in school and social interactions, and even at home.

But, regardless of how difficult it may be to care for children with disabilities after treatment the child will learn how to cope with and manage the signs.

The signs

It's difficult to tell whether your child suffers from an illness or issue without seeing any signs. Here are the signs of ADHD and they are divided into three categories, each having distinct behavior patterns.

Hyperactive-impulsive type

The indicators comprise:

Always seeming to be headed to someplace

You can't sit for too long

can'tplay quietly

excessive talking

scribbling out answers, before getting the full answer

fidgeting or fidgeting or

excessively running or excessive climbing or

Always interfering or obstructing

the difficulty of getting a turn standing in the line

A type that is not attentive.

The indications are:

distraction

Always losing things such as notebooks, toys or even homework

Not paying attention to daily routines

organizational issues

issues with keeping focus on work or other play games

issues with paying attention to the details or committing careless mistakes in other tasks or schoolwork

I am unable to follow directions

Does not enjoy tasks that require mental energy.

apparent listening problems

A type that is combined

A mixture of inattentive and hyperactive-impulsive kinds is extremely frequent

While the task of caring for them can be difficult, it is essential for any parent to ensure that they keep in the forefront of their minds that they aren't poor children. They do not have a motive to be difficult and aren't acting out.

Diagnosis

There isn't any test to identify ADHD however , a diagnosis could be established through a thorough examination. The majority of children who suffer from ADHD will be assessed and treated with the help of pediatricians as well as primary care physicians, others may be referred psychiatrists, psychologists, or neurologists. These specialists can be a huge help in aiding children who is unsure of their diagnosis or if there are other issues, such as depression, learning disabilities, Tourette syndrome or anxiety.

To be diagnosed as having ADHD:

A child has to exhibit behaviors that fall into one of three categories prior to age 12 years old.

The behaviors have to be persistent for at least six months

The behaviors have to occur in a negative way and then affect the child in at minimum two different areas such as friendships, home and school settings, or in childcare environments.

These behaviors are more severe than those of other children similar to them

These actions displayed by the child shouldn't be attributed to stress at home. This is due to circumstances that could lead children to lose their memory or even act out. These include health issue, divorce or move schools, changing homes or any other significant life incident. To ensure that your child is not being misdiagnosed, it is important take a close look at your past and see if any of these events could have contributed to the symptoms you've noticed.

In the beginning your pediatrician will conduct a physical exam, and ask you questions about the medical history of your child such as any signs and concerns and their previous health as well as family health. They will also ask about any medications your child might have been taking, the allergies that the child might be suffering from or other concerns.

The pediatrician can also assess the hearing and vision of the child, so that other medical conditions could be ruled out. This is due to the fact that there are emotional disorders like anxiety, extreme stress , and depression that can manifest as ADHD. Parents are usually provided with a questionnaire that they complete to let the doctor know whether they can rule them from the disorder or not.

Parents should be prepared to respond to a variety of questions concerning the child's growth and behavior at home, school and with the other children. Adults like teachers and nannies should also be considered since they spend a lot of time with children and may be the first to recognize the ADHD signs. It is essential for every participant to be completely transparent and open regarding the child's shortcomings and strengths.

What are the causes of ADHD

The use of vaccines, bad parenting or a child who consumes a lot of sugar or food that is sugar-loaded are not the cause of ADHD.

ADHD is a biological disorder, but they aren't fully discovered. There is no definitive reason for ADHD currently, however, studies are focusing on the genetic and environmental causes. Certain studies have shown that children with ADHD have a close cousin who suffers from the same condition.

Although researchers aren't sure whether this is the cause that is causing ADHD However, they have found that certain areas that are part of our brains five to ten percent smaller in size and activity in children who suffer from ADHD. Researchers have also discovered that ADHD children exhibit altered brain chemicals.

There is also evidence linking smoking cigarettes during pregnancy to ADHD in children. Other risk factors may be severe brain injuries during birth, or low birth weight and premature birth.

A few studies also show that the excessive use of TV by children with attention issues in the near future. Parents must make sure that children under 2 years of age do not need any screen time. Those who are two years old or over should be allowed to use it for 1 to 2 hours per each day, or less.

Treatment ADHD

While this illness has none of a cure for it, it has to be controlled. The doctor will collaborate with parents to develop an ongoing, individual strategy. The main goal is to help the child to develop the skills to manage their behavior, while assuring the members of the family to create a space where this is possible.

The majority of the time, ADHD is best dealt with a mix of medication and behavior therapy. A good treatment plan should include monitoring and regular monitors by the doctor, who may modify the treatment plan along the method. Because parents must be involved in their child's treatment program as well, education of parents is essential in ADHD treatment.

There are certain signs such as hyperactivity that might diminish in intensity as a child grows older. However, problems with attention and organization tend to remain. But, over half of children who suffer from ADHD struggle with their symptoms in their early years of adulthood.

Medicines

There are several drugs that are utilized to treat ADHD which are:

Non-stimulants are wonderful to utilize when you need alternatives to stimulants, but they can be employed in conjunction with stimulants. They are less likely to cause negative effects than stimulants and can last for as long as up to 24 hours.

Stimulants - These are the most well-known medication and have been used for more than 50 years. Some stimulants require a certain number of daily doses, with each lasting for around four hours or twelve hours. There are a few side reactions that can be experienced, like stomachache, irritability as well as a decrease in appetite and sleepiness. However, they haven't reported any long-term effects.

Antidepressants can be considered as a treatment option however, the FDA issued a warning on the subject in 2004, stating that these medications may increase the likelihood of suicide among adolescents and children. If an antidepressant is recommended for treatment parents should talk about it with doctors concerning the potential risks.

The effects of medications on children differ for each child and what is effective for one child might not be effective for another. So, when you are trying to find the correct medication for your child the doctor might suggest medications in different dosages in case there is a different problem that's causing ADHD.

Treatments

Therapy for behavioral disorders

The results of studies have shown that drugs employed to address issues with attention and impulsive behavior are more effective when they are paired with the use of behavioral therapy. The therapy attempts to alter the behavior of the child by:

A system with constant rewards for behavior that is acceptable and harsh consequences for unacceptable behaviour

The child's school and the home environment

Clear and precise instructions and commands

Strategies for tackling behavior for your child

Create a schedule that you can follow. Endeavor to adhere to the same routine every day from the time you wake up until night time. Place the schedule in a spot that the child is in a position to easily see it and be aware of what they are expected to do for instance, when they need to play, perform chores, or do their homework.

Get organized. There should be a designated area where bags or toys as well as clothes are stored on a daily basis. In this way, the child will not be lost or need to look for something.

Get rid of distractions. switch off the cell phone, computer television, radio, and other devices to focus on your work.

Offer a limited number of choices. Give your child too many options to pick from. Limit to only two choices. So your child won't be overwhelmed or overly stimulated.

Change your interaction with your child. - Eliminate lengthy explanations in your conversation and make it short and concise when reminding your child of what you expect from them.

Use incentives and goals. You can write on a paper goals for your child . be sure to reward them for good behavior with the option of a reward. Be sure your goals are achievable for your child. Taking infant steps can be a good option.

Utilize effective methods for disciplining - Although yelling and spanking will not yield the desired outcomes, the loss of privileges or time outs can help your child realize the consequences of their unacceptable behaviour. But, if the child is young, it is possible to be a distraction or ignore the child until they follow through with what you expect of them.

Let your child figure the talents they have. Every child should achieve something they are happy about, so finding out the things your child excels in, regardless of which it may be, can boost their self-esteem and social abilities.

Alternative Treatments

While the only treatment options that treat ADHD that have proven efficient are behavioral therapy and medications, certain doctors may recommend additional treatment and interventions based on the symptoms and needs for the particular child. Certain children may require special educational interventions , such as therapy for occupational disorders, or tutoring.

Other treatments that have been tested and are endorsed by parents are diet modifications as well as chiropractic treatments, Attention training, megavitamins allergy treatment, conventional one-on-one psychotherapy, and visual training. It is worth noting that there is no research-based study that has proved any of these alternative treatments efficient and the majority haven't been thoroughly studied.

Be aware that parents should stay clear of any treatment which claims that it will cure ADHD.

Chapter 2: Signs and symptoms

Life is a delicate task for every adult however if you're always tardy, disorganized, demotivated and overwhelmed by obligations, you might have ADHD. Attention deficit disorder can affect many adults and its many annoying symptoms can impede everything from relationships to your job. However, help is readily available and understanding ADHD can be the initial step. Once you've figured out the problems you can begin to overcome weak areas and begin using your strengths.

The condition of attention deficit is often unnoticed throughout the adolescent years. It was especially common before as not many people knew about ADHD. Instead of recognizing your symptoms and understanding the root of the issue Your family, teachers or even other individuals could have considered you to be as a dreamer or fool, poor-for-nothing or a troublemaker or a terrible understudy.

However there is a chance that you've had the ability to adapt to the signs of ADHD as a child but then you'd run through problems as your demands increase. There are more balls that you're trying to throw at the wall trying to find a job and raising a family managing a family unit, the greater the focus on your capacity to manage, focus and keep from worrying. This isn't easy for anyone, but in the case that you suffer from ADHD it may seem like you're out and out in a way that's unimaginable.

The best part is that regardless of how you feel it may be, the issues of ADHD can be overcome. Through training, support and a touch of innovation it is possible to figure out ways to manage the signs of adult ADHD in addition to turning certain weaknesses to strengths.

For adults Attention deficit disorder typically is not as obvious as in children. Moreover, its symptoms differ for everyone. The following categories highlight the typical signs of adult ADHD. Make sure you can identify the areas where you experience difficulties. Once you have identified the most risky symptoms and signs, you are able to look at strategies to treat the condition.

Focusing and Concentration Problems

Adults who suffer from ADHD often have difficulty being focused and focusing on day-to-day tasks. As an example, you may be distracted by non-material images and sounds, then skipping from one task to the next, before moving on to the next or be exhausted fast. The symptoms of this category are often ignored because they're not as difficult than the ADD/ADHD signs of impulsivity and hyperactivity but they are just as difficult. The symptoms of inattention as well as problems with fixation include:

"Daydreaming" without even realizing even in the course of a discussion

Incredible distraction and a swaying mind can make it difficult to stay completely focused.

Problems focusing or concentrating like when listening or reading

Doing their best to complete tasks, even those which appear to be simple

A tendency to ignore the subtle aspects which can cause mistakes or ineffective work

Insufficient listening skills; difficult time recalling discussions and following notes.

Hyper focus

Although you're likely aware that those who suffer from ADHD have difficulty focusing on tasks that aren't interesting to them, you might not realize there's a second factor: the tendency to become absorbed in tasks that are stimulating and lucrative. This is known as hyperfocus.

Hyper focus is actually an approach to deal with stress to diversion, a technique to block out the confusion. It may be powerful enough that you become completely unaware of what is happening in the surrounding. In other words, you may be so enthralled by books, the TV that is on, or your computer that you forget all about time and neglect the things you ought to be in your mind.

Hyper focus is an advantage when directed to productive exercises, but it could also cause problems with relationships and work when not controlled.

Unorganized and forgetful

If you're an adult with ADHD life can appear to be chaotic and wild. Being calm and composed can be to a significant degree challenging, as can figuring out the relevant information for your current task, arranging the tasks you need to complete, keeping track of the tasks and commitments and managing your schedule. Common signs of complexity and lack of focus are:

Lack of authority (home office, work location, or vehicle is to a large extent messy and confused)

Procrastination tendencies

It is difficult to begin and finish projects.

Constant delay

At times, it is possible to overlook obligations, arrangements and due dates

In constant loss or destruction of things (keys phone, wallet or other documents, bills)

You may not think about how long it takes to complete your assignment.

Impulsivity

If you are suffering from the negative effects of your symptoms during this class, you may have difficulty controlling your actions, comments or reactions. It is possible to act without thinking about the consequences. You could end up imposing on others, making comments or rushing through your assignments without understanding the guidelines. If you suffer from impulse problems patience can be incredibly difficult. For better or worse, you could be swept into situations and land in potentially risky situations. You may have to contend with powerful driving forces in the event you

Sometimes, you interfere with others or speak over them

Do not exercise restraint.

Make comments that are unconsiderate or unconvincing without taking into consideration

Are prone to addiction

Do not act impulsively or abruptly without regard for the consequences

Are you having difficulty in the most socially appropriate ways (for example, sitting but in a lengthy meeting).

Emotional Issues

Many adults with ADHD suffer from severe difficulties with their emotions, specifically when it comes to feelings like anger or sadness. The typical symptoms of adulthood that are enthusiastic and enthralling for those with ADHD are:

Feeling that you are not doing enough.

It's not easy to handle discontent

Clearly irritated and stressed

Frequent emotional or physical episodes

The inconvenience of constantly being up and down

Hypersensitivity to feedback

The short, frequently irritable temper

A lack of self-esteem and the feeling of fragility

No Sleep and Hyperactivity

Adults who exhibit hyperactivity with ADHD may appear the same as in children. It is possible that you are wildly excited and always "on the move" like an engine. Some people suffer from ADHD On the other hand, symptoms of hyperactivity are likely to be less visible and inward-facing as they get more well-established. The typical signs of hyperactivity among adulthood are:

The internal euphoria of the mind or anxiety

Propensity to take risks

Getting exhausted effortlessly

The swooning thoughts

Uncomfortable sitting still; constant wiggling

Longing for energy

Talking too often

Doing a million different things without any delay.

Conditions that can be related to ADHD

Although this is not often the case, certain number of children may also exhibit symptoms of various concerns or issues related to ADHD like, for instance,

Tension disorder is a condition that causes your child to feel stressed and be anxious for a good period of time; it may also trigger physical symptoms, such as rapid pulse, sweating , or wooziness.

Oppositional defiant disorder (ODD) This is characterised by problematic and negative behaviors, particularly toward powerful figures, like individuals, teachers and people

Conduct disorder typically is characterized by a tendency to exhibit hostile behavior, including fighting, taking vandalism, hurting people or animals

Wretchedness

Problems with sleeping - thinking it's difficult to find the time to rest around the evening hours, and experiencing occasional sleep examples

Autism spectrum disorders (ASD) can affect the way people communicate, social connections as well as hobbies and behaviour

Epilepsy is a condition that affects the cerebrum, and triggers recurrent fits of seizures

Tourette's syndrome is a condition that affects the sensor system depicted by a mixture of automatic clamors as well as the development known as tics

Challenges to learning, for instance dyslexia

Chapter 3: Diet For Adhd - Foods That Can Help

Recent studies have shown that the use of prescription medications for ADHD management could trigger numerous adverse effects, including diminished growth, hallucinations insomnia, anxiety, digestive issues, heart ailments and damage to the chromosome (which could lead for cancer). There's been an evolution towards a natural method of ADHD intervention one of which is changing the diet of people with ADHD. What is the ideal food regimen for ADHD?

Diet plays a vital part in treating ADHD and can help in reducing the symptoms. However, there's no one diet that works for everyone. This is due to the fact that ADHD is an atypical disorder. Each person with it requires an individual treatment and is biologically distinct. The most appropriate question could be, what diet that will best suit your loved ones with ADHD?

Adults and children with ADHD are spotted to have nutritional deficiencies. They are deficient in calcium, zinc magnesium, iron, and fat acid (omega 3, 6) within the body. Certain foods like sugar coffee, caffeine, carbs dairy, wheat and other food additives can cause more harm to the patient. It is commonly found that the most efficient diet for ADHD includes two elements that include the nutrition supplementation to compensate for deficiencies in nutrients and the avoiding of foods which can trigger manifestations of ADHD.

Before trying any type of diet to treat ADHD it's recommended that you consult with a doctor to ensure that the regimen is appropriate for one's specific health condition.

Elimination of food items

It is not known if a food item can cause ADHD However, research studies have revealed that certain food items can exacerbate the symptoms of ADHD such as foods with additives (artificial coloring artificial sweetener, artificial flavoring and preservatives) as they can create allergies and enhance the signs of ADHD. Organophosphate is a common ingredient found in non-organically grown fruit and vegetables, can cause short-term memory issues, behavioral changes, and impacts the development of the brain. So, it is best to avoid eating foods that contain preservatives or synthetic ingredients. Also, those suffering from ADHD should consume organic or locally grown vegetables exclusively.

Elimination diets often used by people suffering from ADHD include the gluten-free diet (no carbs from wheat), Feingold diet (no diet with additives) as well as the Casein Free Diet (no dairy products that contain protein).

Supplementary Diet

A great diet to supplement your diet for people suffering from ADHD can be one packed with fruits, legumes, and vegetables. These are because they are high in polyphenols. Polyphenol isn't only beneficial in fighting and treating cancer but also enhances memory, brain's cognition, and the overall operations. It is also beneficial for overall operation. Mediterranean Diet is known to improve longevity, and it's the most effective diet for brain health as well. It's an ideal supplement to a diet for ADHD. But, kids can be very picky eaters. Additionally, the hectic lifestyle makes it difficult to cook homemade meals all the times. If they use the homeopathic ADHD supplements to fill the gap in dietary deficiencies, people with ADHD can benefit a lot. These supplements are rich in omega 3 as well as magnesium, calcium zinc and iron. Studies have shown that those suffering from ADHD gain a lot from when they use natural ADHD supplements.

A diet designed for ADHD children has been specifically created or designed to meet the requirements of children suffering from ADHD. The foods that are suitable for ADHD children have been specially chosen to address the nutritional requirements of kids with ADHD and also to ease the effects certain food items can trigger. The typical diet plan designed for ADHD kids has restrictions on certain foods as well as an established program that must be adhered to of the food items to eat frequently.

Many studies show that certain food items can cause adverse effects on certain children, triggering the beginning of Attention Deficit Hyperactivity Disorder or Attention Deficit Disorder in these children, and aggravating those symptoms that are associated with these disorders. This is the reason diet therapy is believed as a viable alternative treatment for ADHD for children. Consuming the right food choices and avoiding food items that contribute factors to the occurrence of

ADD/ADHD has been proven to offer some relief from symptoms of ADD/ADHD.

Dietary restrictions that may be essential in the successful implementation of the treatment include:

Sugar. Sugar has been linked with the hyperactivity of some children. It's been reported that eating excessive sugar may cause children to have irritable temperaments as well as hyperactive behavior and aggression. The research hasn't found enough evidence to prove that sugar is an influential factor in the manifestation of ADHD/ADD.

Processed food. Research has shown that certain children may have negative reactions to processed food items or those with coloring, preservatives and other additives. Processing foods can increase signs of ADHD in children.

Dairy products. Research has also shown that children who suffer from ADHD are allergic to dairy products like cow's milk. Consuming dairy products may enhance the symptoms that are indicative of ADHD for children. This is why it is suggested that children suffering from this disorder should not consume dairy products.

Foods that are junk. Junk food is bad for children, whether they have or not ADHD. These types of food are not nutritionally beneficial in them. They may be even worse when they are given to children suffering from ADHD since they have the potential to increase the severity of symptoms.

Respecting the guidelines above will greatly help in reducing signs of ADHD. The following food items for children may even yield greater results:

Nuts and ground flax seed. These foods are ideal for children suffering from ADHD and are full of fat acids.

Nutrient-enriched foods. These types of foods are beneficial not only for children suffering from ADHD however, they are beneficial for all people. Foods that are rich in nutrients have properties that can help the brains of children with ADHD to function better.

Omega-3 fats. Omega-3 fatty acids found in foods such as fish and oil that contain very low mercury levels could assist in developing a more efficient functioning of the brain and reduce the onset of hyperactivity in children suffering from ADHD.

It is possible that results won't be brought from a diet change for ADHD children in a matter of hours. It may take some time before you can see results. However, it's worth the effort and time. It's even more effective used in conjunction with other treatments such as herbal remedies homeopathic treatments as well as behavioral therapy and other alternative treatments and supplements.

ADHD and food additives

Over the years, parents have attributed their children's behavior problems and hyperactivity, inattention, and impulsiveness to certain elements of their diets, including the consumption of sugar as well as food ingredients. Over the years, studies have not been able to pinpoint the root of these behaviours which are referred to as attention deficit hyperactivity disorder , or ADHD. However, researchers have identified a number of dietary elements that may contribute to ADHD as well as other aspects that seem to ease symptoms.

Sugar has been a target for criticism due to its image for causing problems with behavior among children for a long time. Many parents believed that excessive sugar in their diets led their children to behave badly and remove sugar from their diets. This strategy didn't work with the majority of children, but it did end up it made parents question the possibility of sugar being the cause behind the child's ADHD. Recent research has shown that sugar does not cause ADHD and hyperactivity among children. it won't cause ADHD even though an eating plan that is filled with sugar isn't an optimal one.

Another element of the children's diet that has been linked to ADHD was the use of red food dyes. These additives to food were extensively studied for their connection to ADHD and even though they haven't been proven to contribute to ADHD red food colorings can cause more symptoms of ADHD in a lot of children. Because of this, experts believe that food dyes which contain red are best avoided for children with characteristics of ADHD to help them manage their behavior.

Certain dietary elements have been proven to improve kids' behavior suffering from ADHD specifically Omega 3 fats. If they have higher levels omega acids than kids with ADHD who didn't supplement their diet, those with ADHD had a better improvement in their behavior.

We're getting a better understanding of what can improve symptoms, and which dietary elements can contribute to ADHD however the precise reason for ADHD for children remains to be a mystery.

Chapter 4: A Complete Variety of Causes and Treatments

The medical profession seems to ignore any single element that could cause ADHD and would prefer to list a variety of aspects that could cause the condition rather.

The reason of the decrease may be due to polygenetic nature. Particularly, those genes that regulate how the brain works with dopamine as a neurotransmitter receptor are believed to be completely altered in children who suffer from ADHD. Other theories could also be based on prenatal alcohol intake and fatty acid deficiencies impaired glucose metabolism, as well as thyroid problems as one of the various possibilities for the cause of ADHD.

With the help of establishing consistent boundaries through behavior management techniques Some doctors believe ADHD symptoms could be eradicated. The top of the listis Sugar is definitely extremely controversial in regards to its adverse impacts on children and the possibility that it could cause ADHD. According to the research you've read about it is possible to be confused about its relationship to the behavior of children.

The Dr. William Crook, a pediatric physician who treated children who were hyperactive for more than 25 years, reported in an ongoing study of five years, in which he interviewed parents of 185 children who were hyperactive and found that the majority of children were negatively affected by their diets. He concluded that their increased activity was definitely linked to certain foods they ate with the biggest culprit was sugar.

Another study was conducted from The New York Institute of Child Development in NYC which involved 265 hyper-active kids. It was shocking since they discovered that 75% of children did not efficiently digest and digest sugar as well as the other carbohydrates that are refined. Further research conducted by the National Institute of Mental Health revealed that the typical rate that the brain utilizes glucose, which is its primary power source for energy is less for those with ADHD than those who do not suffer from ADHD.

When there is a deficiency of blood sugar (also called blood sugar) the body releases a reserve, epinephrine. It is generally referred to as adrenaline. Adrenaline is a hormone which provides the body with an energy boost, which is referred to as"a "sugar surge" also known as a "sugar spike". The body is then pushed to the state of hypoglycemia (low levels of blood sugar) because it is eating less or in the opposite case, taking in excessive amounts of sugar. People suffering from reactive hypoglycemia could be suffering from a metabolism issue which causes an over-secretion of adrenaline.

Another Yale study that successfully tested how sugar affects blood glucose levels and levels of adrenaline. The study found that level of adrenaline for children was 10 times more than average for 5 hours after the consumption of sugar. She says that studies that show a weak connection between sugar consumption and behavior are typically inadequate and poorly executed.

Children who are hyperactive are most sensitive to salicylates that naturally occur along with phenolic substances. Salicylates are typically employed as food preservation agents and can be found in the manufacturing of aspirin. It was found that food additives could cause hyperactivity following the investigation of more than 1,223 instances where additives were directly associated with behavioral issues. Artificial colors, salicylates and artificial flavors found in our diet have been shown repeatedly to be the primary cause of the excessive activity of children.

The issue was mentioned as early as 1940 that there had instances of food dye sensitivities aspirin, aspirin, and the naturally occurring salicylate compounds found in vegetables and fruits. It was discovered that the majority of a vast group of children with hyperactivity were tolerant to hyperallergenic diet. When they were on the diet, some of the kids' behavior changed to normal. The most frequently triggering substances were artificial food colorings and preservatives.

A healthy diet for children with hyperactivity was highly advised based on the assumption and scientifically proven hypothesis that food additives such as artificial colors, flavors, and preservatives can cause hyperactivity. If they were placed on strict diet, free of any additives, children significantly improved and began to exhibit normal behavior.

In a trial lasting six weeks in which the children were put on a diet free of synthetic food. Parents of 155 children reported notable improvements in their behavior. However, they observed that when artificial colors were incorporated to their diets, the behavior of their children deteriorated. The more the food coloring that they were consuming in their food and drinks, the longer their "bad behavior" was in effect.

It was also discovered that by removing these reactive food items, such as those containing artificial colors and food additives as well as artificial colors, the ADHD symptoms of restlessness, irritability, as well as a variety of other negative behavior were drastically diminished. Through PET images of brains, researchers can examine how much glucose specific areas of the brain use. Examining the brains of those who suffer from ADHD there are specific regions of the brain that have shown significant reduction in the utilization of glucose as well as a decrease in brain metabolism. Researchers are currently looking to determine the root of this decrease in glucose metabolism among those with ADHD.

Another known neurodevelopmental disorder that resulted in ADHD symptoms has been linked to Fetal Alcohol Syndrome (FAS). FAS is typically not caused by excessive consumption of alcohol during pregnancy and FAS children typically have lower birth weight, impaired intelligence, as well as other physical deformities. Children with FAS show the same level of hyperactivity, and the same low levels of impulse control and inability to focus like children with ADHD.

Many recent studies have led researchers to conclude there's a connection between thyroid dysfunction and ADHD. It was observed that as high as 75% of children who suffer from a condition that is known by the name of "generalized thyroid resistance" are also afflicted with ADHD symptoms.

People who have thyroid resistance experience decreased glucose levels in cells, which is now known to affect the brain's metabolism. The impaired glucose metabolism is directly connected to ADHD in the event that the decreased brain activity is located in the brain area. It's the reason we have the ability to pay attention , and is also responsible for our behavior.

Thyroid problems can be the result of stronger synthetic chemicals such as PCBs as well as phenols and excess histamines. Deficiency of fatty acids can be connected to thyroid dysfunction. The majority of brain tissue is made up of phospholipids, a type of fat that originate through essential fatty acids. numerous studies have identified the essential fatty acid (EFA) deficiency in a number of hyperactive children.

A study recently that was published within The American Journal of Clinical Nutrition found a link between blood levels of omega-3 and ADHD in boys as young as. EFAs play a significant role in neurotransmitter function , which is crucial to the transmission of neurotransmitters as well as the proper development of nerve cells.

Recent studies have also demonstrated that psychostimulants actually cause brain atrophy. This conference, which included 29 experts from the nation who were experts on ADHD found that there was, at present not enough evidence to conclude there is evidence that ADHD can be a medical problem.

Traditional Treatment:

The typical dosage is a small dosage (5 up to 10-mg) and increasing it each month in line with a decrease in those ADHD symptoms. Drugs that cause side effects are monitored. are frequently switched out if adverse effects are too intense or if no obvious changes with the behavior of the child.

The most popular medication available today to treat ADHD can be found in Ritalin (Methylphenidate hydrochloride). Also, there is a brand name drug such as Concerta which has identical chemically. It acts as a central nervous system stimulant which increases the production of neurotransmitter (dopamine) or, that is to say, very similar to what cocaine.

The side effects may range from the abnormally fast heartbeat, blood pressure fluctuations abdominal pain and weight loss, nausea, palpitations and skin irritation, skin rash, dizziness, drowsiness and fever hair loss, headaches, joint pain and insomnia, as well as nervousness as well as loss of appetite. Tourette's syndrome to psychotic reactions.

Another medication that is commonly prescribed that is used for ADHD can be Adderall as well as Adderall XR (d-amphetamine as well as amphetamine combination). The drug inhibits the re-uptake and release of neurotransmitters and prolongs their action and reducing metabolism.

Common side effects include blurred vision, headaches constipation or diarrhea weight loss, nerves, seizures, irritability and euphoria. Other symptoms include insomnia dry mouth, fast heartbeat, dizziness or a decrease in alertness, decreased appetite nausea, and an irregular heartbeat.

The drug was pulled off it's market Canada due to its link to heart problems in young children. However FDA did not issue a warning in Canada. FDA only issued an "warning" to the USA.

Other medications could also be prescribed for example, Trazadone to aid sleep through the night for children or an anti-anxiety medicine in the event that they begin to show Tics or twitches (Paxil, Wellbutrin, Klonopin).

Sometimes, the fluctuation of medications can cause the child to have hallucinations and suffer from "mood changes" and then they are recognized as being suffering from Bipolar Disorder (it is now a well-known diagnosis for children) and then an anti-psychotic medication can be prescribed (like Depakote or Zyprexa).

The Naturopathic Treatment

There are many reasons that have led a lot of doctors to doubt the validity of ADHD. The first is the severe side-effects from the medication given to children. In addition, there is increasing evidence of little or no long-term improvements in students' academic performance There is also the issue of what conditions that diagnose the ADHD.

It seems that common child behaviors, or the reasons for "failing" to complete their chores or schoolwork, aversions to and isn't interested in homework, or is unable to wait for their the next turn, can be used to determine if a child suffers from ADHD. There is also the realization that psycho-stimulations don't cure the root of the behaviours they simply provide the patient with a permanent "band aid" to treat the disorder. But, a variety of naturopathic or alternative treatments may actually solve this "disorder".

A new study in clinical research has demonstrated the efficacy of nutritional interventions in comparison to conventional psycho-stimulant treatments. These results strongly support the efficacy of supplementation with food treatments to improve the self-control and attention of children suffering from ADHD as well as suggest the treatment with food supplements of ADHD could be of similar effectiveness (if not better) as Ritalin treatment.

In the wake of theories about food-related triggers for hyperactivity have been discussed, there have been many different theories that support an edgier diet as a remedy. The diet is referred to as an "elimination diet" because it involves the process of eliminating all food items which contain synthetic or natural salicylates.

Natural salicylates comprise fruits and vegetables like apple, almonds and plums. Prunes, prunes and strawberries. They also contain pickles, cherries, apricots as well as raisins, grapes oranges, peaches, cucumbers, tomatoes and vinegar.

Synthetic salicylates refer to all foods which contain artificial colors as well as artificial flavors such as sodium bisulfate, benzoic acid sodium nitrate and potassium

Sulfites BHA, BHT, MSG Butylene Glycol, tartrazines.

After a child's behavior has normalized, which could take between 4 and six weeks, food items can be gradually introduced into their diet , and then closely monitored to determine their impact in the behavior of the child. It is suggested that all members of the family follow a similar diet in order to provide the child with complete moral support, since the diet could be extremely restricting.

Foods with adverse effects on the health of children include Artificial colors as well as preservatives. Oranges and grapefruits, eggs and MSG processed dairy products and milk, grains (not entire grains) sugar.

It is also suggested that an eating plan high in calcium, magnesium B12 (increases energy, eases anxiety, and improves concentration) and omega-3 fish oils (contains DHA important in brain health) protein (stimulates cognitive alertness) and zinc (important in the proper functioning of neurotransmitters) as well as vitamins C and B6 (important in the immune system and metabolism functions) Pycnogenol and extracts of grape seeds (two herbs that boost blood flow to the brain) and probiotic (helps maintain healthful bacteria that reside in digestive tract).

The drugs used to treat ADHD can cause serious negative side effects such as psychosis and can cause manic as well as schizophrenia-related episodes. When these side effects occur doctors don't stop taking medication, but they prescribe more medications and diagnose the child as suffering from depression or an antisocial personality disorder. They treat the child with mood stabilizers, antidepressants or Narcoleptics. It is not uncommon to find children using up to five different medications that can cause a myriad of additional side-effects. There is a expression "Meds on meds is madness on top of madness."

Many studies suggest the benefits of increasing protein intake to boost serotonin levels, which is calming to children who are hyperactive. It is also recommended to consume large amounts of B vitamins, with an emphasis in B6 (pyridoxine) as well as vitamin C, as well as essential fat acid (EFA's).

In a research study that was conducted, high doses of B6 were administered to children who were hyperactive for 7 weeks . This was followed by seven weeks Ritalin followed by 7 weeks of placebo. The dose that was high of B6 proved to be the most effective treatment which raised blood serotonin levels, whereas Ritalin did not.

It is also suggested it that EFA supplementation of between 1,000 and 1500 mg of capsules in the evening time are consumed in the morning and in the evening. Certain children showed better results to the evening primrose oil if it was massaged into their skin. This is because quite often, children who are hyperactive may suffer from poor digestion.

In the Summary:

Recent research supports a the use of natural remedies for ADHD which is a condition that was previously thought to be an unnatural response to environmental triggers (if it is true that an illness exists). There is a lot of evidence for dietary triggers that trigger ADHD behavior of hyperactivity and inattention. They are mostly due to sugar consumption and food additives, defective metabolic process of glucose (sugar consumption) and fat acid deficiencies.

Parents have the option of choosing to the treatment they provide their children. They do not are required to put their child on the risky psycho-stimulant medications. They could be exposing themselves to a long-term habit of dependence on drugs for their children and also labeling the child with a disorder that could have long-lasting implications if they believe there's something "wrong" in them.

The best method for treating of ADHD might require a bit more time and effort from the parents when it comes to restricting their child's diet, however, the advantages of this approach are significant. The root of the child's behavior is discovered, and then nipped in buds, and not hidden by treating the symptoms by using harmful drugs.

The most recent research focuses on the use of multivitamin and multi-mineral supplements, herbal as well as getting rid of all the toxins from the food chain, such as foods colorings and additives and heavy metals. All seems to have a significant impact on the reduction of a child's ADHD symptoms, but without the risk of negative side effects.

Recommendations for Treatment Summary:

* A thorough assessment by a naturopathic doctor to determine the

presence of a food allergy and a dietary assessment to determine if a nutritional deficiency is present.

Eliminate any processed food which contain artificial ingredients such as aspartameand Butylene Glycol, potassium Bisulfate sodium nitrate and potassium, benzoic acid, sulfites BHA, BHT, MSG and tartrazines from the diet.

Eliminate natural salicylates like tomatoes, cucumbers, cherries and almonds. Grapes, Apricots, apples, berries and raisins, as well as citrus fruits, peaches, plums and strawberries. vinegar, and pickles out of your diet.

* Include a vitamin or mineral supplement each day: EFA supplement containing omega-3 EFAs such as those found in EPA Fish Oil capsules Extra B-complex (120 or 150 mg daily) and zinc (20 -30 mg daily) as well as Selenium (100 or 200 mg per day) Vitamin C (1,000 to 2000 mg, daily) and calcium (1,000 1500 to 1,500 mg daily) Magnesium (300 to 500 mg daily) or take

the an oil of evening primrose (2,000 or 3,000 mg daily in 2 doses).

* Calming herbs like St.John's valerian, wort, or skullcap to lessen the signs of hyper-activity and irritation.

Chapter 5: Medical Cure

Traditional Treatment

The use of prescribed medication is frequently utilized to reduce or eliminate signs of ADHD however, there is no evidence to support its efficacy.

As the condition has grown more recognized and more medications have been added to the market to combat it.In certain instances there is no doubt that medications can be beneficial however, in many cases it has been discovered to cause unpleasant and dangerous negative side effects.At the best, medicines may help alleviate some symptoms but other symptoms persist. Of course, if the medication ceases it will also stop any relief that may be found.

The fact that medications that help treat ADHD are able to cause harmful unwanted side effects can suggest that conventional medicine isn't always the most effective solution.There are two kinds of treatment for ADHD which are stimulant and non-stimulant.They are able to affect the quantity of dopamine released in the brain.Dopamine is a neurotransmitter that stimulates the brain for the point of action or motivation. It may help sufferers focus more effectively while reducing their hyperactivity. These include Ritalin Dexedrine, Ritalin, and Adderall. Although these are effective remedy for many, other people could be severely damaged by their use.The negative side consequences of stimulants that can be observed include:

*Difficulty sleeping

A loss of appetite or stomach upsets

*Palpitations

*Dizziness

*Tics

*Depression

* Bad temper

*Irritability

*Headaches

*Restlessness

Even if the side effects were to be ruled out it is not clear regarding the long-term physical and emotional impact.ADHD is a relatively new issue and medications, which can be prescribed in treating it could cause other issues within the body.

Research so far has been insufficient to be able to discount detrimental effects on brain development.Stimulants are open to being abused and teenagers can and do use them to give them an unnatural boost.They might also be responsible for precipitating psychiatric problems because they are altering the chemical compounds of the brain.Stimulants have also been found to be the cause of cardiac arrest in those with a pre-existing heart condition.

If someone who taking the stimulant medication is experiencing any of these symptoms it is recommended to contact your doctor immediately:

*Paranoia

*Chest pains

*Hallucinating

*Shortness of breath

*Fainting

The non-stimulant drug Strattera does not do as well but does come with lower side-effects.It is not able to affect dopamine that is found in the brain however it does affect a different chemical in the brain known as norepinephrine.It can also be used as an anti-depressant , however it is discovered to be less efficient as stimulants.It is still able to cause adverse effects, including:

*Nausea

*Headaches

*Vomiting

Ailment in the abdomen

*Sleepiness

*Moodiness

*Dizziness

It's not surprising that the interest in the use of natural cures has stimulated in the hope of avoiding uncomfortable and in some instances, potentially dangerous side-effects.It may be even proven that damage to the brain caused by these medications is disproportionately reduced in rewards and respite.

In the next section, we'll look at how medication are able to be eliminated and replaced with natural remedies.What can you integrate into your daily routine, often quite easily, to eliminate any symptoms associated with ADHD or at least reduce them to the extent that conventional medication promises?

Chapter 6: Causes of Adhd

In reality the actual causes of the disorder aren't known However, research has revealed possible causal factors. The causes of the disorder are interconnected and range from genetic and environmental. In some instances, other causes like illness or brain damage, as well as food intake can contribute to the disease. We'll take a look at a few of these causes to aid in understanding the condition more clearly.

Genes

The condition can be passed down by parents who have genetic mutations that trigger the condition. Furthermore siblings of those who suffer from the disorder are three to four times more susceptible to the disorder than which no member of the family is affected by the disorder. Genetic factors may also determine if the disorder can be treated in childhood or persists into the time of adulthood.

According to studies conducted by researchers, children who carry one particular kind in the ADHD gene was identified to have weak brain tissues that were affected in regions. The differences between brain regions affected and non-affected were not significant, and recovering processes improving the condition as the child matured. As an adult normal brain development and normal thickness was that it was likely to recover while the symptoms decreased.

Further research is being conducted to determine the genes that be most likely to being the cause of the disorder among individuals. Finding the genes that are involved can assist researchers in limit the development of the disorder among patients who have been diagnosed with the disorder. In addition, this will aid in the development of more advanced or efficient treatment options.

Environment

Research has revealed a link between smoking cigarettes and drinking alcohol in pregnancy and ADHD for children. Additionally, children exposed to large amounts of lead might be more susceptible to developing the disorder. Lead metal is commonly found in paints as well as in plumbing sites.

Substances like nicotine alcohol, and lead are extremely toxic and can be harmful to brain tissue. If children are exposed to these substances during the beginning stages of development and growth, they could develop ADHD. But, these experiences don't create different brain development among young children and adults with ADHD.

The environmental trigger that could trigger the disorder are pesticides. A study conducted by pediatricians observed that children producing urine that contained excessive levels of pesticide wastes were more susceptible to ADHD. Chemicals used in pesticides are organophosphate. Women with high concentrations of organophosphate were at greater risk of carrying a child who has an ADHD condition. It is possible that there is a link of connection to pesticides, and ADHD however, enough evidence is not available to back up the findings. The best method to protect yourself from ADHD is to consume organic varieties of fruit and vegetables as they contain fewer pesticides in the course of growing.

A lot of video games have been discovered to have a negative effect on college students and children with issues with attention. It is due to the constant stimulation both of these causes students uninterested. This is why bad parenting is often blamed for the children being raised with poor behaviors, taking into consideration that a bad parenting approach can cause ADHD behavior.

However parents, you can't be held accountable for the disorder. If you establish consistent boundaries on behavior, you can make use of consequence-based tools, or rewards, to establish a clear expectations which can help reduce the severity of the symptoms. Also, being in a family that is stressed and with parents who might not be supportive of ADHD because it is a severe illness and demanding lifestyle can worsen the condition.

Low levels of Omega 3 fatty acids

The findings also suggest that children with the ADHD disorder could be suffering from insufficient levels of Omega-3 fat acids present in bloodstreams. It isn't yet clear whether the insufficient amount of Omega-3 fatty acids can contribute to or worsen the symptoms. But supplementing with Omega-3 like taking fish oils could help reduce the problems associated with ADHD in some children. Studies have found that taking 1 Gram of Omega-3 for approximately 3 to 6 months is moderate to strong efficacy on ADHD. There are other studies that suggest similar outcomes, particularly in instances when

Omega-3 fats were mixed with zinc and magnesium.

A long-term study focusing on the impact of Omega-3 in a model animal of the disorder known as Attention deficit hyperactivity disorder has identified gender-specific differences in the manifestations of the disorder. These findings have led to the idea Omega-3-rich fatty acids could be a secure method of tackling the disorder. Other aspects like gender are also a factor in these instances.

Brain Damage

Brain injuries could cause Attention deficit hyperactivity disorders particularly for children. The brain injuries may be the result of circumstances like stroke, trauma or brain tumors, among other serious illnesses. However, only a tiny fraction of children suffering from the condition may have suffered brain injuries.

Sugar Diet

There are many who believe the consumption of refined sugar with one of the reasons for ADHD disorder. To confirm this, one study gave an infant group with sugar-sweetened soft drinks and another group of drinks artificially sweetened. The study did not find any differences in the level of activity between the two groups of children. While sugar isn't proven to trigger hyperactivity in every child but some children suffering with ADHD exhibit hyperactivity following drinking sugar. It is therefore recommended to check your child's behavior to determine if sugar makes them hyperactive or not.

Food coloring and additives

The research also has found an association between consumption of certain food addictions such as artificial preservatives and food colorings and hyperactivity. Children who consumed these addictives were observed to be more hypersensitive however, they had different levels of hyperactivity. The study found that the use of food coloring or other addictive substances can increase hyperactivity by around 10. Other research has revealed that eliminating these substances from children who suffer from ADHD condition can help reduce the severity by 33-50 percent.

Based on these research findings the conclusion is that just a small percentage of children are susceptible to the adverse effects of artificial flavorings or additives. However, determining what children are susceptible to the disorder was not easy. Therefore, more research-based evidence is needed to validate the findings and discover the mechanism by which the additives cause hyperactivity.

Food-related diseases or Allergies

Many studies have shown that food intolerances , or allergies can trigger the development in ADHD symptoms. The causes of these allergies may include the inability to digest protein that is common the cause of celiac disease. Limiting your child's exposure to certain foods they may be allergic to may serve as a means to manage the condition. This is because sensitivities to food or nutritional deficiencies can play a part in ADHD.

Complications during Pregnancy

Do you realize that a challenging pregnancy can result in children with ADHD? The aforementioned issues may be present as soon as when the fetus is growing in the uterus or even later, targeting the brain of the baby when the baby is born.

The most frequent problems that can arise in children includes high blood pressure during pregnancy and bleeding, particularly prior to the birth. Other signs could include the baby being in the womb longer that anticipated and taking longer to go through labor. There may be additional serious complications that can impact the baby's oxygen supply during the delivery.

The diagnosis of ADHD

ADHD Diagnoses for children

The treatment for this disorder will be based on several factors that will determine if it's evident or whether it persists into adulthood. Additionally, as kids with different characteristics may exhibit different personality traits, levels of energy or temperaments it might not be prudent to connect all of these to ADHD. There may be a range of signs among children between the ages of 3 and 6 years old, such as hyperactivity or impulsiveness. Parents and teachers will be quick to recognize differences in behavior expectations.

Therefore, it is crucial to run a number of tests before concluding that your child might be suffering from ADHD. It's usually a matter of visiting an accredited pediatrician to evaluate your child. Be aware that certain pediatricians will assess your children on their own and others might recommend an individual child to a mental health professional. Both share the same objective of determining whether the symptoms that the child is experiencing are a sign of ADHD.

A few of the indicators to be aware of include:

The child may have difficulties with learning

If there are any issues with hearing or vision that are not apparent.

If there is any ear infection , it may be a contributing factor of hearing difficulties, in addition to ADHD

The child may be suffering from medical issues that may affect the child's behavior or way of thinking

What might be causing medical issues, like undetected seizures.

If the child could have been affected by a sudden major change like the death of someone, loss of employment of parents or divorce of parents

If depression or anxiety could be involved, it is best to seek out the source.

The results of these tests are then compared to medical or school records to find numerous indicators. These findings can aid the medical professional in determining the presence of abnormal or restricted indications. Other family members with whom you know your child could also be of assistance like babysitters or coaches, as well as other adults.

A medical professional should determine the possibility that the symptoms could help in making informed decisions about various matters, including:

If the actions are permanent and influence everything in the life of the child

If the behavior is continuous or only occur in isolated instances, it could be caused by other triggers,

The behavior could be observed in various locations or in certain places, like at home, in the school or on the playground

Are the problems specific to your child or are they similar to those of your child's peers.

In all of these stages of evaluation The expert monitors the child's behavior in various scenarios. Additional tests can determine the way your child behaves in social situations, his or her health condition, intelligence as well as the level of learning. If the results of these tests prove that your child suffers from ADHD the child is likely to be diagnosed with the disorder.

ADHD Diagnostics in Adults

If ADHD persists, you should have it evaluated by a licensed mental health specialist. The majority of adults who exhibit symptoms of the disorder comprise approximately 60 percent of kids who exhibit ADHD behavior into adulthood.

For older adults, depression can be behind many negative behavior issues, including depression, relationship issues and work-related issues, as well as drinking and drug abuse. It is essential to make a proper diagnosis in order to make sure that the primary source of the problem is discovered and it becomes easier to deal with the issue.

In the course of diagnosis, the physician may consider whether the problem began in childhood and then progressed all way through adulthood. This would be the basis to determine the root cause of ADHD. Another important aspect is studying your behavior's patterns. This can be done by speaking to your closest family and friends. In addition, you'll need to take a physical examinations and a variety of physical tests.

If you have determined that you are being affected, you will require counselling to understand the dangers of the disorder in your daily life. Additional disorders like anxiety and depression could also require attention based on the way you behave.

ADHD as well as Anger Management

If you suffer from ADHD regardless of whether you're an adult or a child it is likely that you'll be unable to control your temper, and will likely have anger-filled outbursts. In particular, kids might have angry outbursts when they are being with friends, doing their homework, or just being with the family. Adults can also experience anger when dealing with daily activities that may be challenging to living a peaceful life.

Anger Management in Children

The most effective method to help your child to manage anger is to use exercise , as it can aid in reducing the effects of anger. Exercises help improve the neurotransmitters' actions in the brain, which in turn helps to promote healthy living. Opportunities like joining an organization, participating in martial arts, or other sports activities can greatly help.

Another option is to talk to your child about methods of defusing anger since language can be effective in calming anger. The use of language that is motivating can cause your child think more carefully and reflect on the situation. Studies have shown that children who suffer from issues with language usually behave angry and recklessly.

Adults with Anger Management

The following suggestions are useful in managing anger among adults:

The primary step in this process is to determine the reasons or triggers that cause anger by highlighting situations that trigger your anger. When you are aware of these triggers it is important to avoid them and discover how to breathe and relax.

The other option is to not dwell on negative thoughts that cause irritation and replace negativity with positive thoughts.

If you take into consideration the consequences that anger can bring about it is possible to minimize the negative consequences by understanding how to manage your anger effectively.

Being positive is also an approach that is recommended to think of several positive alternatives to the causes of anger.

Appreciating yourself can be very beneficial since it gives you a reason to improve and help less people. This increases the chances of acknowledging your achievements and increasing self-esteem.

Chapter 7: Dietary Changes, Restrictionsand Supplements and Nutritional Support to Treat Adhd

According to several research studies ADHD occurs in those with an ancestral experience with the disorder. However, many environmental triggers and dietary factors have a role to play in it. Studies have shown that synthetic sweeteners and refined sugars preservatives, chemical food additives cause nutritional deficiencies that can gradually lead to ADHD.

While there are medicines for ADHD however, they come with several adverse negative effects. The majority of ADHD medication eases symptoms by balancing and increasing the levels of various hormones involved in the development of ADHD. Drugs like stimulants such as Adderall and amphetamine, which aid in focusing and reduce distractions, as well as non-stimulants such as bupropion can help reduce the hyperactivity. However, they usually come with numerous side effects, including insomnia, mood swings as well as loss of appetite and heart conditions.

A recent Australian study has revealed that taking medications to treat ADHD doesn't cause significant changes in the way that people deal with attention issues and behavioral problems. Additionally, those who used medication to treat ADHD were experiencing elevated levels of diastolic blood pressure , and were self-esteem-shy. With these concerns in mind experts on the subject and health care professionals find that it is best to cure ADHD by using natural methods.

The most efficient and safe methods to combat ADHD is to alter your diet, take nutritional supplements, and alter your eating habits to the healthier. In this chapter, we will provide information on the various methods of improving the condition through improving your diet as well as using natural supplements.

Dietary Restrictions

There are certain restrictions on diet that if you begin doing so will have a positive impact on your child. Based on the Mayo Clinic, certain food colorings and preservatives increase the amount of hyperactivity, which is why it is important to beware of them. Be sure to examine the ingredients of packaged and processed food items prior to purchasing them. Also, avoid products that contain the following preservatives and colorings.

FD&C Yellow No. 6: This yellow sunset coloring is typically found in soft drinks, cereals confectionery, icing, candy and breadcrumbs.

FD&C Yellow No. 5 Sometimes referred to as tartazine this coloring is often used in pickles, cereals yogurt, and bars of granola.

D&C Yellow No. 10: This yellow quinolone coloring can be found in sorbets, juices and sorbets as well as in smoked haddock.

It is also known as sodium Benzoate can be found in dressings for salads, carbonated drinks and juices for fruit.

FD&C Red No. 40: This red color is typically used in medications for children as well as soft drinks, frozen cream , and gelatin-based desserts.

These colors and preserves typically cause irritation and hyperactivity that may trigger and even exacerbate ADHD. In addition, it is recommended to avoid the following allergens that could trigger allergies:

Chemical preservatives and additives such as butylated hydroxytoluene, as well as butylated hydroxyanisole , which serve to ensure that the oil in a product fresh are not recommended for use in. Preservatives like these are also present in processed food items like chipping gum and potato chips dried cake mix, instant potato mashed cereal, potatoes and butter.

Chocolate, eggs, milk and peanuts can trigger allergies in certain people. If your child is allergic to any of them or any other fooditems, be sure to stay away from it.

MSG as well as Aspertame are two of the ingredients found that are present in the majority of processed foods that are used in the present and should be kept to a minimum.

Furthermore, numerous studies have shown that ADHD is usually caused by eating sugar in huge quantities. Consuming foods that are high in sugar triggers a child's hyperactivity that causes and can exacerbate ADHD. To reduce the symptoms and ensure that it does not get worse the problem, stay away from drinks, juices and other foods that contain sucrose, dextrin and maltodextrin and malt syrup as they are all types of sugar that increase levels of glucose that in turn trigger the issue.

When your child is able to stay from these food items gradually introduce foods that contain the following nutrients into the diet of your child, since these nutrients ease signs of ADHD and help to combat the issue effectively.

The nutrients you need to Treat ADHD

The following nutrients aid in restoring those hormonal balances (mainly an increase in dopamine levels) that cause and can aggravate ADHD Therefore, make sure that you incorporate foods rich in these nutrients to your diet. It is recommended to select foods that are organic and meats that are grass-fed whenever possible. This reduces the risk of exposure to chemicals in the food produced using standard methods that can be toxic and accumulate inside our cells. They must be cleansed from the body so that we can see the huge benefits in repairing ADHD symptoms.

Iron Magnesium, Iron, along with Zinc: Zinc regulates the levels of dopamine. This is a neurotransmitter essential in the development of ADHD. Zinc levels are insufficient and are associated with low level of focus; therefore when you increase the amount of food consumed by your child that is that are rich with zinc, it will will gradually improve the condition of your child.

Iron is a different nutrient that is required to make dopamine. Therefore when their levels of iron are low, it's likely that the body isn't producing enough dopamine to combat the effects of ADHD. Furthermore, magnesium is essential to make neurotransmitters which improve concentration and concentration. Magnesium is also known to calm the brain, so the consumption of foods high in magnesium may help to address the issue.

The three minerals are found in grass-fed meat, grass-fed poultry, nuts and seafood. When your child eats a greater amount of foods with natural ingredients that are high in these minerals, make sure that they are taking wholefood multivitamins or multimineral supplements containing iron, as they increase the level of these minerals in the body, allowing them to manage ADHD more efficiently.

Omega-3 Fatty Acids: Omega-3 fatty acids are vital for brain and nerve cell function. A study carried out by researchers from the Goteborg University, Sweden found that daily doses of omega-3 fats aids in reducing ADHD symptoms and signs by up to 50 percent. They also enhance brain function and reduce inflammation which can further reduce ADHD symptoms.

Omega-3 fatty acids can be present in salmon, sardines tuna, tuna, and nuts seeds. Make sure your child eats food items that are rich in omega-3 fats. You can also supplement your child's diet with omega-3 fatty acid-based supplements like Nordic Naturals, MorEPA, Barlean's Omega Swirl, Omega Rx, OmegaBrite and Green Pasture.

Vitamin B: Studies have shown that increasing the intake of B-vitamins can reduce aggression and eases ADHD symptoms. The most B-vitamin-rich foods include: legumes, orange juice liver, dried beans cereals fortified with B vitamins eggs chicken, milk, and milk-based products. Also, you should add B-vitamins supplementation to your child's diet , such as Bio-Strath. It is recommended to consume 50 mg of food that are high in B vitamins to slowly eliminate ADHD.

If you're adding these essential nutrients to your child's diet, you should make space for the following supplements and herbs, as they can help alleviate ADHD symptoms.

Supplements and herbs

Ginseng and Gingko These two herbs are referred to as cognitive activators that is to say they function as stimulants, similar to ADHD drugs, but without off-shoots. They can help you become less distracted, less hyper, and more focused.

GABA (gamma-aminobutryic acid) It is an amino acid known for its calming properties that helps to ease ADHD symptoms. A dose of 100-200 mg of GABA consumed three times a day can do wonders in overcoming ADHD. But, make sure you consult your doctor prior to taking GABA as it might not work for everyone.

Pycnogenol: It is an extract extracted from French pine tree that has been proven to increase hyperactivity, improve concentration and attention as well as improve motor coordination in the visual sense. The herb is rich in antioxidants and polyphenols that help protect brain cells from free radicals and enhance cognitive abilities. Pycnogenol is available as a supplement however, only take it after consulting your physician.

Rhodiola Rosea: Created from the Rhodiola Rosea plant that grows in the Arctic region, this natural supplement boosts your attention as well as your accuracy and alertness. It is recommended for kids over 12 years old and adults as it may over-stimulate young children.

Picamilon is a unique combination of gamma-aminobutryic acid (GABA) and B-vitamin Niacin This supplement improves the flow of blood to brain and enhances concentration and alertness. This helps to reduce ADHD symptoms.

Make the modifications to your child's diet and, as you continue to do this, you'll notice significant changes in their behavior. The best way to slowly overcome ADHD is to be aware of how different foods that your child consumes impact their attitude and behaviour. Note what you notice in a diary.

Remove slowly one food item from their diet , and substitute it with one of the foods that help ease ADHD together with a supplement, and observe what happens. If you see better results then introduce additional ADHD comforting food items to the diet of your child.

For supplements, consider two to three supplements each for 4 weeks to determine which one is the most effectively for you. Choose the one or two that work for them the best. It is advisable to speak with your physician prior to beginning any supplement to ensure that they can advise you to take into account your health of your child and any other medical issues they might have.

Alongside dietary adjustments In addition to dietary changes, you can treat ADHD with other approaches to treat ADHD. We will look into this further in the next chapter.

Chapter 8: Handling Adhd through Structure And Routine

The struggle with ADHD even though it can be a burden for parents, isn't an unsolvable problem. The truth is that solutions are at hand and the disorder is manageable. One among the best treatments and solutions to ADHD is to provide and keep a regularity. Like the name suggests it's about maintaining some type of order and structure at home as well as in school.

The key is determination.

Willpower is a crucial factor in establishing routines. Parents often give up at any time perhaps because of frustration or exhaustion , or either. But aren't all children , even those who suffer from ADHD worth the effort put in by parents and their caregivers? It's crucial not to quit. Begin today if you have been unable to do so. Set up your family routines and make a commitment to maintain these routines. Although the path to creating and maintaining routines for children with difficulties with attention may be difficult, there is a an end to the tunnel. Beginning parents may see every day a constant fight, However, routines are likely to work when they are used not just as strategies to change behavior but rather as an integral part of daily life.

Consistency

It is crucial to establish routines starting in the early morning, when your child awakes and continues through the time in the evening when sleeps. The most important thing here is coherence. The same thing that is performed at 7:00 am on Monday should also be carried out on Tuesday, and through Sunday. It doesn't necessarily mean that the child is living like they was in a military school. It is important to include enjoyment into the child's daily routine.

The advantages of structure

There are many advantages with routine and structure. Psychologists and experts in parenting stress that having a structure is essential particularly for children who have attention issues. Generallyspeaking, having a regular schedule will help them to keep track of their time at home as well as at school, and can lead to better behavior.

They also help ADHD children to become more effective and to function effectively. Schedules give a sense of security and help children develop positive behavior and efficiency. They understand that order exists in a chaotic world, and that rules or certain limitations must be adhered to.

Thirdly, when everyday activities are planned and monitored regularly, the process becomes more planned and reliable. This can lead to better management. This is advantageous for the caregivers and also for the person who is being looked after.

Fourth, as the child is able to follow the implementation of an established schedule, the child gets an awareness of direction as the child gets used to daily chores. The child is able to predict the things to expect. They know, for example when it is 10:30 am the child must take a trip to the sink to wash his hands using soap, wipe them with the hand towel, then place himself at the table and eat breakfast. Then, the routine becomes mechanical and routine once they have develop into a routine. In addition, caregivers adopt similar routines and find things simpler to handle. Through routines, parents can free themselves from unnecessary stress since they don't need to rush to find the next event for their child.

Fifth, regular routines alleviate stress on the part of parents as well as the child, as they both are aware of what is expected at a specific moment, even though there are ADHD children who have to be reminded of their routines.

Furthermore, because daily activities are planned that the child is focused on one task at one time. This prevents overburdening the child, and can help those who suffer with anxiety disorders in addition to ADHD.

Be sure that the tasks of the day are prominently displayed for both the child and you to observe. For children who are visual learners, drawings or illustrations of certain activities can aid in recalling the routines. For instance, a picture of a faucet such as a faucet, for example, will remind the child that must wash his hands at a specific time like after lunch.

Being able to have routines allows you to enjoy peace and tranquility at home as well as in a schools. It also provides the family members the opportunity to fulfill specific roles and help in the correct functioning of the individual suffering from ADHD. Since each member of the family is involved in activities together, the sense of family is built and the identity of the family established. The child discovers that their older brother is the one who takes dishwashing to the sink, and that the big sister cleans the table after meals.

Whatever your schedule are, ensure that you do not neglect or abandon the idea of keeping a well-organized life for your own sake as well as to benefit the child suffering from ADHD. At the end of the day you'll reap benefits that include greater productivity for both you as well as your child, improved relationships with your family, and improved overall health, in addition to. In the Journal of Family Psychology has revealed the fact that all children are likely to have better health and display good behavior when they are raised in a home with rules or routines.

It could take months or even years to get your child comfortable with the structure, but your child and the entire family will be worth the effort. Additionally, the advantages will last for a life time. If you haven't started to set up routines, it's time to begin. The next time you're ready to give up consider reconsidering. Make sure to keep the resolve to remain committed to keeping the structure in place and to remain consistent in the execution of assignments, no matter how challenging and exhausting.

Chapter 9: Treatment Options

In general, the first line in treatment of ADHD sufferers is medications.These drugs are made to aid ADHD sufferers concentrate and restrict their impulse-control. The drugs prescribed for ADHD typically are known as psychostimulants. They are considered controlled substances, which means you have to possess current and valid prescriptions and refills are closely controlled.The most commonly prescribed stimulant drugs are:

Ritalin

Adderall

Concerta

Daytrana

Focalin

Metadate CD

Dextrostat

Dexetrine

The medications are intended to increase the production of certain neurotransmitters which are believed to stimulate or activate the impulse control and attention centers of the brain. They aid the brain in paying attention to the child and help to reduce the hyperactivity and impulsivity that are associated with ADHD. These stimulants can cause serious side effects, however, and must be administered in a carefully monitored environment.The most common side effects are headache, insomnia, and the loss of appetite. There are also non-stimulant drugs that are approved to treat ADHD. Although they aren't as effective, these drugs are often used when the effects of stimulant medication are a source of concern or get too severe.

The most common non-stimulant medicines include:

Wellbutrin

Kapvay

Intuniv

Strattera

Alongside medications in addition to medication, various techniques for managing behavior have been shown to be effective in treating ADHD symptoms. ADHD. For children, the therapy of parent-child interaction that teaches parents to demonstrate the desired behavior while reducing the unattentive or impulsive ones, is frequently utilized successfully. Training for parents is another approach which teaches parents to identify and treat issues, and after the child has become older enough, cognitive behavioral therapy helps a child regulate their behaviors by knowing the way their thoughts and emotions affect their behavior. Talking with your child's teacher will help them succeed at school, regardless of their disorder. Methods like daily report that targets specific behaviors have been proven effectiveness. The development of social skills can aid in ensuring that children behave better when playing with other children. Additionally, therapy sessions for families can aid parents and children deal with the difficulties caused by the child's behavior and needs.

A lot of children are able to overcome their symptoms before they enter the middle school age, when symptoms start to diminish or disappear. However, some children suffer from symptoms that could affect their lives as they grow older. The symptoms of inattention tend to persist throughout adulthood, but not hyperactive or impulsive.Many adult who exhibit the inattention symptoms are likely to take their medications and treatments into adulthood.

Parents often ask these questions when their child is identified as having ADHD:

Did I do a bad job as a parent causing ADHD in my child?

No. ADHD is caused by chemical imbalances in the brain, particularly in the region of the frontal lobe. An unorganized, abusive or chaotic family life can make it harder for children to cope with those symptoms and could lead to more aggressiveness.

Can my child overcome ADHD?

Many children will eventually get over the diagnosis they were given, but the symptoms can persist throughout adulthood, and require for them to require expert help in managing them.

Can medications negatively impact the brain of my child?

Based on research studies conducted on ADHD sufferers, most of the drugs that are prescribed to treat ADHD do not have long-term impacts on the structures in the brain. Children have been safe taking stimulant medication for a long time but, like all medications, it is important to constantly monitor them for any adverse effects that could be adversely affecting them.

Does medication impact my child's ability to learn?

It Can.ADHD kids who take medication tend to focus better and are more prepared to make more of their school time more than they did they were before.

Does diet aid in the treatment of ADHD?

There isn't any research-based evidence yet to establish a link between the effects of diet and ADHD however, diet may play an important role in any of the behavioral disorders in both adults and children. A few studies have revealed that fish oils can reduce symptoms of ADHD.The studies have shown that ADHD patients who use fish oils may experience greater relief than those taking Adderall, Ritalin, and other drugs that are commonly prescribed to ADHD patients.

Certain foods and drinks may have a negative effect or worsen some symptoms related to ADHD.Stimulant drinks like sodas, coffee and certain fruit juices with excess sugar or stimulants, such as caffeine, should be resisted or avoided.Foods with a high amount of sweets or artificial substances can increase hyperactivity and make it more prominent.Recent research has also revealed that stimulants may cause certain behavioral issues for both adults and children. Ritalin and Adderall along with other stimulants have been associated with bipolar disorders, psychosis Manic depression, bipolar disorder, and schizophrenia episodes.More research into the relationship to diet and its effect on mental disorders like ADHD are being conducted.

Do the minds of ADHD sufferers different from other?

Yes. Brain scans are known to reveal differences in the size of brain regions that are focused on the impulse and attention control centers.

Chapter 10: Strategies for Controlling Symptoms and Staying Focused

There's hope for those with ADHD in adulthood, no matter how chaotic your life gets and no matter how overwhelmed and frustrated you may feel. With support, structure, and a personalised set of self-help techniques Learn how to stay organized effectively control your schedule, gain charge of your finances, enhance your job performance, and improve your social abilities.

If you suffer from ADHD it can be overwhelming. Everything from making sure you pay your bills on time and managing the demands of family, work, and social obligations can be overwhelming. However, it is possible to stay focus and transform chaos into peace. Through self-help strategies, you can be more efficient, well-organized, and in control of your own life. It will also improve your self-esteem.

Adult ADHD can cause challenges in every aspect of your life, from organising at home to achieving your full potential at work. It could be detrimental to your health as well as your professional and personal relationships. The symptoms can cause extreme procrastination, difficulties meeting deadlines, and an impulsive attitude. You may also be concerned that family members and friends aren't understanding what you're going against.

There are many ways to get the issues with ADHD in check. You can enhance your habits every day, learn to recognize and apply those strengths and create techniques to help you achieve greater efficiency, enhance efficiency, and connect better with other people. It won't happen overnight However, it is possible. These strategies for self-help in ADD/ADHD need perseverance, practice and, perhaps the most important an optimistic attitude.

Tips to get organized and managing clutter

The most prominent characteristics of ADHD disorientation and inattention can make organizing the biggest issue that those suffering from the disorder confront. If you are a sufferer of adult ADHD and you are a parent, the idea of organizing regardless of whether at home or at work could cause you to feel overwhelmed.

But, it is possible to break down tasks into smaller pieces and use an organized method of organization. Implementing different routines and structures, and making use of tools like calendars for the day and reminds you will be able to keep your organization in check and manage the clutter.

Establish a structure and tidy routine and maintain them

To arrange a room at home, office or home Sort your belongings into categories and decide which items are essential and which should be kept or put away. To keep yourself organized begin the practice of writing notes and lists. Keep your new structure by following regular routines for your day.

Create space. Consider what you require in a day-to-day basis and then find storage bins or closets to store things that you do not. Set aside specific areas for items such as bills, keys, and other items that may easily be lost. Get rid of things you don't use.

Make use of a calendar application or a day planner. The use of a good day planner or calendar on your phone or computer will assist you in remembering deadlines and appointments. With digital calendars, it is possible to schedule automatic reminders so that you don't forget important dates in off your calendar.

Use lists. Use notes and lists to organize regularly planned tasks, projects deadlines, appointments and tasks. If you choose to use an everyday planner, be sure to keep the entire list and notes in it. There are many choices to use your phone or computer. Find "to do" apps or task manager.

Get it resolved Now. You can stay clear of confusion, forgetfulness, and procrastination, by filing your papers and tidying up mess or answering phone calls right away now, not later in the near future. If you can get a task accomplished within two minutes or less take it immediately instead of put it off until the future.

Take control of the ADHD paper trail

If you suffer from adult ADHD The most prominent cause of your disorder could be a mess of papers that is scattered all over your desk, kitchen or office. Spend a few hours setting up a paper system that is a good fit for you.

Create an organization system for filing. Make use of dividers, or separate folders to store different kinds of files (such such as receipts, medical documents or income reports). Label and color code your files to make it easier for you to find the information you require quickly.

Handle the mail daily. Take a few minutes every day to handle mail, usually when you get it into your home. It's helpful having a specific area to sort the mail , and sort it out, either to throw it away, put it in a file or take action on it.

Go paperless. Reduce how much paper to manage. Get electronic statements and invoices in lieu of printed copies. Also, you can reduce junk mail by abstaining from the Direct Marketing Association's (DMA) Mail Preference Service.

AdultADHD self-help myths

It is possible that you have false beliefs about how much you can aid yourself in dealing in adult ADHD.

Myth That medication is the only solution to my ADHD.

The truth is that while medication can assist some people in managing the symptoms of ADHD however, it's not a cure or the sole solution. If it is used the medication should be used along with other treatments or self-help techniques.

Myth: Having ADHD signifies that I'm lazy, or incompetent, and therefore I'm not going to be capable of helping myself.

Fact: The consequences of ADHD could have resulted in people describing your behavior in this manner but the reality is that you're not in a state of demotivation or lack of intelligence. You are an issue that stands out of the way of regular functions. In reality, those who suffer from ADHD typically have to come up with extremely creative methods to overcome their condition.

MYTH: A doctor will solve all of my ADHD issues.

The truth is that health experts can assist you in managing symptoms of ADHD However, they're only able accomplish a certain amount. You're the one who's living with the issues, and you're the person who will be the most effective in beating them.

Myth: ADHD is a life sentence that will always cause me to suffer from the symptoms.

Fact: Although it's certain that there is no cure for ADHD but there are things that you could do in order to minimize the difficulties it causes. When you are used to employing strategies to aid yourself, you might discover that managing your symptoms become second nature.

Chapter 11: Various possible causes of Adhd

In the last few years, diagnoses and cases of ADHD are steadily increasing. As per the American Psychiatric Association, at five per cent of American children suffer from ADHD and The Center for Disease Control and Prevention estimates the figure at 11 percent in 2011. The numbers continue to increase as experts question whether external causes could be the main cause for ADHD for kids as well as in adults.

Do chemicals actually trigger ADHD?

The science suggests that it may be a contributing factor. Everyday toxins we find in our food items and in the surroundings are toxic chemicals in personal care products, and even machines could be a major contributor to the increasing number of ADHD cases throughout the years.

Infants and children are susceptible to chemical exposure that is toxic even when they are in their mothers wombs. This is the reason pregnant women are not advised of using any kind of drug or alcohol since these poisons can have a lasting effect on the brain as well as the health of the newborn.

The Learning and Development Disabilities Initiative (LDDI) has released its first-ever report that identifies the chemical populations that members of the disability and learning population are exposed. The report is titled "Mind, Disrupted: How toxic chemicals may affect the way We think and who we are."

The report states that these elements can be a contributing factor to ADHD:

1-Genes that are passed down in the family can influence how ADHD develops. ADHD

2. Non-shared environmental variables like birth complications

3 Environmental factors like the toxins that come from chemicals, fluoridated and chlorinated water from the tap

4-Foods that contain pesticides and insecticides

Five-Growth Hormones, Antibiotics and Meat and Poultry

6-Highly processed food items containing artificial flavors

7-Artificial preservatives and colorants

8-Overuse of prescription drugs

Toxins from chemicals FLUORIDATED AND CHLORINATED TAP WATER

The latest research released by The Lancet of Harvard The Lancet talks about the levels of toxic substances and how they contribute to the rise levels of autism, as well as ADHD.

The study was carried out in collaboration with the Harvard School of Public Health (HSPH) as well as the Icahn School of Medicine at Mount Sinai (ISMMS) says that in addition to pollution from the environment, drinking fluoridated water also contributes to increasing incidence of behavioral and cognitive issues. In the year 2006 Harvard carried out and released research highlighting the detrimental effects of fluoride as a "developmental neurotoxicant'. The current review examines 27 additional studies using a technique known as meta-analysis. The Harvard researchers claim it is the result of a "silent epidemic that is being ignored by the press and studies have largely ignored.

It's simple that fluoride, pesticides metals, herbicides and radioactive isotopes as well as GMO food products are all contributing to an neurotoxic mixture that builds up in the bloodstream and sometimes even gets beyond the blood brain's defenses. While the body attempts to defend itself against the harmful chemical compounds, they ultimately get absorbed by organs and bones, which can cause brain tumors, cognitive impairments as well as birth problems.

Fluoride is known to transfer through the placenta. Despite this fact, the authorities are not yet able to speak out.

FOODS CONTAINS PESTICIDES, INECTICIDES and Herbicides

It's a fact that pesticides pose a threat to the environment , and more damaging to one's health. The more difficult truth to accept is that these chemicals are introduced into our bodies through food. If we consume foods that contain pesticides, insecticides or herbicides, these chemicals get kept in the colon and slowly contaminate our bodies. An organic apple, for instance, has more than 30 types of insecticides and herbicides. The pesticides remain in your fruit long after washing.

These chemicals are connected to cancer but also Alzheimer's disease as well as birth defects and, of obviously, ADHD because they have the potential to cause damages in the brain, reproductive system, as well as the body's endocrine system. Chemicals that are passed from mother to child during pregnancy affect the development of the brain of the infant and can be detrimental when the mother is nursing the baby. Although a non-organic fruit might not cause harm, eating foods that aren't organic over time can cause an accumulation of chemicals which can cause illnesses and disorders. However, despite numerous research which have proven the harmful consequences of insecticides, pesticides and herbicides, organic food is still incredibly expensive, and no regulation is in place to limit the production of foods using these chemicals.

GROWTH HORMONES AND ANTIBIOTICS IN POULTRY AND MEAT

Presently at present, the FDA is currently approving at least six steroids to be used in 'food animals'. These hormones and antibiotics can help animals grow more quickly or produce more meat. For instance, dairy cows are have been treated with bovine growth hormone (fBGH) to boost the production of milk by cows.

According to alternet.org, the USDA's Food Safety & Inspection Service (FSIS) detects potentially harmful antibiotics each week in animals including penicillin, neomycin, as well as sulfa medications.

ARTIFICIAL PRESERVATIVES and COLORING

Additives to food and GMO ingredients are also known to aggravate ADHD symptoms. Beware of additives like Blue #1 and #2 in food coloring, as well as Green #3 Orange B, the red color #40 and #3 the yellow color #5 and 6 aswell with sodium benzoate which is preservative. These chemicals hamper the body's ability to eliminate toxic substances that are foreign to it and consequently can cause adverse effects that can cause behavioral disorders in the brain.

Highly processed foods with artisanal Flavors

The USDA claims that food coloring is safe , however numerous recent and previous studies have revealed that it can cause hyperactivity among children. Following the time of Dr. Benjamin Feingold's research in the 1970s about the role in the 1970s of synthetic colorings as well as hyperactivity among children using food dyes has been subject to controversy but there hasn't been any consensus regarding the severity of the danger. Joel Nigg co-authored a 2012 study that analyzed the effects of coloring additives and their impacts on hyperactive behavior of children. He found that certain children displayed extreme behaviors while others displayed moderate to moderate hyperactivity. Research has also demonstrated that hyperactivity decreased by having these synthetic colorings eliminated from diets that were restrictive. Niggs insists that this is likely because cutting out the processed food items is a better option and provides better results for children suffering from ADHD.

The overuse of PHARMACEUTICAL DRUGS

Monitoring the Future Monitoring the Future (MTF) program has monitored the behaviors of high school and middle school students and concluded in 2008, 2.9 percent of the 10th graders and 3.4 percent of 12th graders used the drug methylphenidate. Methylphenidates help boost neurotransmitters in the brain this is why it's beneficial in the treatment of ADHD depression, anxiety and anxiety. However, teenagers use the ADHD drugs as 'cognitive enhancement agents'. These drugs, like Adderall, Vyvanse and Ritalin can cause other adverse effects, like sleep disturbances, restlessness and anxiety. For adolescents who weren't diagnosed with ADHD in their early years The use of these drugs can result in a behavioral change that could result in adult ADHD.

GUT DYSBIOSIS and ADHD

In the book earlier we discussed the author Dr. Dr. Natasha Campbell McBride's work about Gut as well as Psychology Syndrome and how there's an evident link between diet we consume and ADHD. The author Dr. Mcbride states that the link with our gut and our psychological and neurological issues is unquestionable. It's a simple theory and is completely logical. If the balance of good bacteria versus bad bacteria is the digestive system becomes a mess it is the condition known as 'gut dysbiosis.' The bad bacteria produce toxins that eventually weaken our immune system and put our bodily functions out of sync. The toxins cause loss of the intestinal liner, which can cause various digestive issues one of the most significant is the stress on the nervous system, leading to ADHD and depression, sleep disorders, and more.

What is the gut's link to the brain? Based on Professor Dr. Michael Gershon, our gut is thought of as the second brain'. Our second brain is covered with numerous neurons that are all essential in the functioning of the brain. Our second brain determines our moods, emotions actions and reactions. when our gut is in turmoil there are mood disturbances and neurological issues develop. Serotonin is often called the happiness hormone comes taken from our gut. Dopamine, which aids in focus as well as motivation, attention, and focus comes from the gut. This is the reason why research has shown that issues with the digestive tract can lead to inadequate absorption, which can lead to imbalances in nutrition and nutrient levels which can lead to the amplification of symptoms of anxiety, depression and ADHD.

Chapter 12: Misunderstood

"To be exceptional is to be not understood." I have read The work by Emerson (1841) Self-Reliance for the first time in my college. Emerson mentions Pythagoras, Socrates, Jesus, Luther, Copernicus, Galileo and Newton as people who are not understood. Being distinctive, having unique ideas and being unique and not going with the flowand not conforming to conventions is not just a reason to be not understood, but also a sign of excellence, such as the above examples show.

There are numerous instances of individuals who were thought-provoking but considered crazy due to their concepts that ended up being as a hit. It is common to not understand or respect someone who has a different viewpoint. We generally want people to have normal thoughts or think thoughts that align with our own. Often, those who think in freestyle, do not follow a pattern, or are innovative are viewed as insane, or even insane.

We have heard about Galileo Galilei, who proposed the heliocentric theory in opposition to the doctrines from the Catholic Church that claimed that earth is at the center all of space and time. Galileo observed the stars with his telescopes and observed the evidence and began to discuss his findings at a time in which a differing opinion was not just controversial, but also a heresy (Andrea 1974). Nowadays, anyone who proposes an idea that is new won't be put in the dungeons, however there's still a lot of practices that are not able being challenged.

Many children who are diagnosed with ADHD don't have an illness. They are often misunderstood as to be geniuses. The world judges what it doesn't grasp. Its Old School will probably continue believing that being intelligent is equivalent to being an Straight "A" students. They will think the fact that not being attentive to classes means attention deficit. Schools are free to believe whatever they like. Beliefs don't change facts. The Catholic Church was unhappy with Galilei's theories however, it was an established fact, the same way Galilei himself said: "Eppur si muove." In the same way, no matter what the old ideas are, they won't alter the fact that children are brilliant, even if they're wrongly interpreted.

ADHD is an advantage and not a disadvantage

ADHD includes the reality that's not evident to the casual observer. Many of these children are geniuses. Try it. When you next are having difficulty using your electronic device, consult your son or daughter to resolve the issue for you, regardless of whether you have an ADHD diagnosis. Modern children have an increased capacity to comprehend the world they live. Our intelligence was used to create our world, and they utilize it to understand their own.

ADHD is a personality that is often misunderstood with a diagnosis. But, it's not always lead to success as many people starting with parents, pursuing the schools, psychologists and even pharmacists struggle to make them normal people. The obstinate guardians and educators struggle just like the Catholic Church did against Galilei.

The truth is that the kids of today have a lot of potential. If given the right opportunity, they could change the world. Ken Robinson gives a very excellent example of the possibilities in "The Element" (2009). It was in Death Valley, California, in 2004, it was rainier than the previous years. In the spring of 2005, the entire surface of Death Valley came to life with vibrant, fresh flowers. This was an event which had never happened before and caught the attention of a lot of people.

Similar to what happens to pupils who attend the older School. Perhaps they are dormant because they don't have the conditions that allow them to develop. When they get the conditions they need, they'll achieve their full potential.

It is an unprecedented moment. There has never been a time in the history of mankind such a large number of great thinkers are involved in a battle against the conventional. The modern-day geniuses are most likely the only ones with the capability to deal with the ever-changing technological advances.

In every classroom, we have minds that are different. They are more creative than we do, as their minds are overwhelmed by a myriad of information that wasn't readily available at the time. They're not afraid create a hypothesis and justify the idea with fervor. Perhaps this moment we're holding an idea that was conceived by an individual who was struggling in school. He did not complete their homework, did not listen to their teachers and who failed their tests.

Albert Einstein has been analyzed by contemporary psychologists to establish a diagnosis like schizophrenia, dyslexia or autism (Wolff and Goodman). If Einstein had lived in the present it is likely that he would be classified as Autistic and would be diagnosed with an intellectual disorder.

Einstein himself stated that the process of remembering words, texts and names gave him a lot of challenges, and he's known as to be a genius. However, whenever scientists are depicted as mad in a manner, it's a bit similar to Einstein's. This is the way people act when they don't comprehend what's happening around them. they evaluate it and then label it.

Einstein had a remarkable mind but only about 15 good hours per day utilize it. According to me, Einstein did not have time to expand every aspect of his life or we wouldn't know his name. That's one of the ways that geniuses work concentrate on their tasks and do not think about the surroundings. This is how they can make their work for the world and it's also how technology was born.

With them, the world is now a brand new location where we can live in different locations simultaneously by using ICTs. I am employed with Chihuahua, Mexico in the morning while working at Taylorsville, Utah in the afternoon using the internet. I'm able to accomplish this and many other activities because of those imaginative minds that were always a little bored at school when they were youngsters.

We require more Einsteins even if they're not focusing on the classroom. It is actually necessary for them to be to be thinking about something other. It is time to not believe about being distracted as somehow negative. If we claim that they have a limited attention spans, we're not right. They have a higher concentration span than people who don't achieves anything notable and are extremely driven by their ideas, be it drawing, sports or playing an instrument, watching, or transforming the world.

There were other people who experienced similar problems as Einstein while they were at school. Some of them are known for Thomas Edison, who got expelled from school due to the fact that his teachers believed that the school was not able to learn, and those of the Wright Brothers who never graduated from high school.

In addition, when we read the biographies of people who have succeeded who's names we hear constantly the same thing, it's always clear that they had a head start of their peers in school. I'm discussing Bill Gates, Steve Jobs, Mark Zuckerberg (Tech-Fac, 2013) and many more who achieved success in their lives (Dodgson 2017, Dodgson).

In the near future I wouldn't be shocked to see the teachers of the past, who pressure parents to administer medication to their children so that they are still, purchase an invention, or employ products or an application developed through one of the "ADHD" children.

We require people who dream. Without them, there would not be cars, planes computers, smartphones, and social networks, in addition to thousands of other helpful inventions.

It's a good idea to locate a school that has an educational program that is focused on the discovery of children's strengths and demonstrating possible ways to use those talents throughout their lives. It's great to show them how they are able to make significant contributions and need not be waiting until they are old enough to make a difference.

It would be fantastic to be able to support their philosophy regardless of whether it's distinctive. It's absurd to attempt to make everyone exactly the same and then to label those who do not conform to the norms as sick. In the Old School, it is often an unrealized dream. The majority of the time, it takes advantage of the talent of students as it is trying to force them to change, the truth is that they're more successful than they were.

Focus on a Different Focus

Let's imagine this scenario that a doctor an engineer, artist, an electrician, a writer as well as an astronaut bodybuilder, teacher and an engineer are stranded in an isolated island the duration of a year. Let's say that because of their intelligence and combined abilities they manage to be able to survive. After returning to civilization, they will be interviewed by numerous reporters. Are they all telling the identical story? You should take for a second to consider this question prior to reading the next paragraph , which contains my thoughts.

They all have an entirely different story since they perceive the world through the lens of what they're. This is how they've been doing all their lives, starting when they were young. All of them had abilities and talents that allowed them to become the people they are today. In the beginning the electrician, with his lack of knowledge about aircrafts, is likely to look for cables or devices in the wreck of an airplane or ship in order to try communicating or create tools. The astronaut will recognize the starry skies and be able determine their location. The engineer will speak about the things he discovered as well as the structures he constructed and the doctor will talk about the tools he used to treat his illness, and the artist will sketch a canvas depicting beautiful sunrises and the author will write a book on the adventures where he is the hero.

The same happens to children. They are exactly what they are from the time they're young. If we aren't able to identify the person they are, that's our issue, however they are actors, soccer players firefighters, athletes, gamers YouTubers, teachers, or doctors. They'll always concentrate on what they enjoy, regardless of whether we agree with them or not. If they are able to do things for a living they don't love it will be on us.

Are our focus on the things we love a problem? In the context of ADHD this is a part of the advice we offer. However, think about it this way: there is only one attention available not two. That means that we are able to only concentrate on one thing at the moment. We don't like spending time doing things that waste our time, and neither do children. If you don't want going to church shouldn't attend. People who don't enjoy read don't. People who don't like Math do not. People who don't like History simply don't.

Children have their own passions. If they are interested in engines, they'll probably become mechanics. If they concentrate on building houses, they'll probably become builders If they enjoy sports, they'll probably be a part of thatpassion, and when they dance, they are developing through their love. They are developing and gaining confidence in themselves until they are told by an adult that they have to sit down and read books and write pages in the face of threats and criticisms.

Neuroplasticity and ADHD

One of my teachers once said it is because language mirrors our mind, possibly quoting Chomsky. However, there are different ways to learn about the brain. The development in the study of Neuroplasticity provide us with additional knowledge about the functions of brain. In the past we believed that the brain wasn't in constant motion. We used to believe that the brain couldn't be wired in adulthood, that adults wouldn't learn new things as damaged brains couldn't create ways to create new neural networks (Rivers 2014).

The advancement of knowledge about the human brain is leading to new treatments and treatments for clinical situations. However, if we consider Neuroplasticity to the diversity of life, we can claim that nature has provided us with an extremely effective tool that is full of potential. The brain has more capacity to learn than any other tool in our in our lives. Thus, an individual has the freedom to choose the things to learn. We are entitled to decide what we're going to utilize our brains to do. Adults often criticize the interestsand focus of others particularly children.

However, we shouldn't be afraid. Children who are hyperactive learn a variety of activities at different levels of their lives. Children who tend to be "obedient," and that only engage in a few things, even if they score high marks may not be developing as many brain regions of the brain. They could be not using as much of their potential since they're following what is taught to them and are not applying their creativity and initiative in their daily life.

The brains of hyperactive children are used frequently and if that's enough, they continue around trying to utilize their creativity to resolve the problems of being not understood. The issue is that kids who are hyperactive who are typically highly creative, aren't permitted to explore their fields of interest. As a result their brain development could become stuck if they do not discover a way to stay over the conflicting demands of their parents.

Kids who are hyperactive are often imaginative and spontaneous. But, Neuroplasticity teaches us that it is also possible to reverse. Traditional education can work. It prevents them from being innovative, from talking about their thoughts, or from growing their skills, which will not be useful to the economy , according to the opinions of the older teachers. Teachers need to be aware of the ways in which Neuroplasticity operates and how the development of the brain happens through the learning of things they like, not things that make them afraid and anxiety.

It also shows that individuals can acquire various things during the process of maturing and growing. As adults or adolescents, people may enjoy learning new things that they resisted when they were young. I've seen instances of this in my personal family. My son, Hiram, didn't like math in elementary school, however, during high school, he discovered an interest in Algebra as well as Calculus. He got so adept at it that he started tutoring his classmates in the evenings after school.

The understanding of Neuroplasticity can be extremely useful to those who don't know the capabilities in the brain children with hyperactivity are equipped with. The brains of hyperactive kids can actually sense and process information with great intelligence and in a highly practical way. They process a great deal of information every day.

Our view of intelligence that restricts our ability to perceive the things they are. They don't only learn by listening. They utilize all the senses. ADHD is far of being considered a psychological disability. Their brain is as strong as any other in the universe, and they don't require any additional dopamine stimulation since their brains are able to handle enough natural stimulants.

Success

What's the goal of school? Being successful? Being a part of the economy in the global market? Being able to provide for the family? Being able to purchase a large house and new vehicles? Being able to afford the necessities? Perhaps it's all of these plus a lot more. I am of the opinion that success is things that are different for everyone according to our objectives. But, in either way it always boils down to money.

Teachers tend to believe that having a degree will earn you money which is why they lecture so hard and believe that they're helping students by being strict and uncompromising. But, it's not necessarily tied to school. There are many different ways to achieve success. I have met people who graduated from college but have no job, and wealthy people who have no formal education.

There's a guy in my neighborhood who didn't attend school. Name is Juan Quezada. Google the name. His art is all over the globe. The artist is Mexican ceramic artist. He is from a poor place, in a small rural area which would have most likely disappeared had it not been for his work. At the time he came into this world,, odds were against his. There was no way anyone could have imagined that he would be a contributor to anything. But, he was able to earn money from his work. His talent and creativity enabled him to achieve that. Furthermore, unlike other business managers who hold secrets to their success secret and do the opposite. He taught his local community how to trade. Thanks to him, hundreds of tourists come to his small neighborhood in Mata Ortiz and his gallery each day to purchase his merchandise.

The past was when success could be directly linked to education. However, nowadays the world, there are numerous things to think about. There is a lot of competition that exists and there are a lot of choices for children to decide to be successful in their lives.

The way that schools are constructed do not guarantee their success. Teachers and administrators should not act as if they could have been. There's a better possibility of obtaining work, with someone else, earning the smallest amount feasible. This is what large companies usually do. They employ specialized employees with degrees, and provide them with enough for them to remain afloat, without investing in their future to make money as if then they'll leave and the company would lose a key asset.

Schools don't teach children or teenagers to be financially intelligent in the way that Robert Kiyosaki so eloquently explains this in the book Rich Dad, Poor Dad (2011). Kids who are hyperactive, on contrary tend to take on a job for themselves and start their own business. As is the case for Juan Quezada, who could possibly be a leader in the company if he earned an education, or become successful by making use of his talent as he did.

It's not a method that is suitable for all. That's why creativity is an vital element to cultivate, as is determination, energy, innovation and confidence in oneself. However, this isn't the curriculum taught in schools, it's what schools are taught.

In conclusion I'm not trying to say that the school system is unimportant, I'm just saying that it's obsolete. If a new curriculum is developed, it could be accessible to everyone rather than just handful of children. It could help teach financial literacy creative thinking, confidence, as well as other vital factors that are required for the ever-changing world. It is beneficial for schools around the globe to revamp education in accordance with the current demands.

There are signs everywhere when we pay attention. Kids are eager to learn and they're willing however, we continue insisting on old-fashioned methods. I was struck by the eagerness a child is to learn after I returned from work and I noticed one of my kids who was always struggling in school. He was lying on his stomach, playing the computer. I said hello and he smiled in return, but did not look at me. He was focusing on his task, so I sat near him, and tried to disturb him in the least way possible.

I began to ask questions regarding his movements on the screen. He always responded without looking at me , but I observed that he became attracted by the attention and began to explain the process he was using with great details and enthusiasm. He was participating in a sporting game, selling and buying players, and even negotiating while preparing to play in the playoffs. He was looking through the stats of players and was analyzing whether they would be a good purchase. He even wanted my opinion about specific players. He was actually a clever thing that demanded concentration.

In the real world , there are people who do what the man was doing to earn a living, and they earn a lot of money because generally, they're the proprietors of a business and in this case is the NBA. I was convinced that he was learning about business via games on video. I remember getting up and thinking that he was learning something that is very valuable. He was in fact training to become CEO.

Chapter 13: Treatment for Adhd or

Add In Adults

There are a variety of methods to use. A majority of people look for medication. They may not be aware or do not realize that every illness can be addressed with self-help or assistance from a loved one. The only thing you require is determination and faith. The next chapter focuses on the treatment of adults that is natural , and provides the opportunity for a holistic growth.

Self-help

When you are fully aware of the issues posed by ADD/ADHD it is possible to make significant adjustments to your life with the help of organized strategies based on the knowledge you have of the condition. Many people suffering from the ADHD have discovered novel and beneficial methods to overcome their symptoms and live an enjoyable and successful life. Instead of viewing these issues as a burden , take the situation in your way and utilize them as an advantage. The outside help can be sought in the event that self-help doesn't result in. In most cases, you can take steps to help yourself conquer these symptoms and bring them under control.

Get active and eat healthy

A vigorous exercise routine must be adhered to regularly. This allows you to burn off the extra energy and aggression positively and also soothes and relaxes your body. Consume a selection of healthy food items and reduce your sugar intake. This can help reduce mood swings.

Sleep well.

A restful night's sleep that lasts 7-8 hours is extremely vital to your health.

Practice better time management

Make dates for all tasks, including minor tasks. Utilize alarms and timers to track time. Make breaks on a regular basis to ease stress and avoid getting your work done. This will allow you to perform your work in a more efficient and efficient way.

Make sure that you create a safe working environment

Make frequent lists and employ techniques such as color-coding and reminders to your yourself. This ensures that you are in a position to manage the time you have and your resources a logical way. If you can, take on your work that you are interested in and be involved in more group tasks.

Outside help for an ADULT with ADD/ADHD

If symptoms of ADD/ADHD continue to be present after self-help strategies to manage the symptoms, you may want to seek help from a professional. Adults with ADD/ADHD as children, will be capable of benefiting from a range of therapies that can help such as classes in soft skills as well as support groups and group therapy.

Professionals with training in ADHD/ADD will be able to help you overcome your issues and overcome your obstacles without a lot of difficulty:

- Helps you control your impulsive behaviour

- Helps you manage time better

- Improves your money management skills

- Enhances your ability to organise

It can help increase your productivity.

- Helps you deal with your anger and stress

- Helps you communicate better

Chapter 14: A Few important Tips

for Adults Living with Adhd

Many people with ADHD believe that they are constantly being burdened by the demands of daily life. That is why they typically get up from their beds feeling like they are one step behind in their daily routine. Due to that feeling, they are able to feel as if they're constantly trying to catch up throughout the day then they go to bed and feel that they didn't get all of their work done.

If these suggestions given below are followed this feeling of rushing about but not getting anything done is not likely to arise as frequently.

Here are the best tips:

Not so quick

People with ADHD often appear like they're working at a high speed. If this is the person you are familiar with, take a break for a short time and then try to complete the same thing in a more sluggish manner. In certain instances it is necessary to slow down before speeding up! If you slow down just to a certain extent and consider the steps required to finish the task, it'll be accomplished much more easily and less stressful.

Do your best to take care of yourself

Adults suffering from ADHD tend to place everyone before themselves. This means that they have not enough time for them. The time that was available has been taken by others. The person in this situation cannot make a difference until they can save the time they need to themselves.

Know Your Personal ADHD The Signs of ADHD

ADHD can have different consequences on individuals with different characteristics. It is important to know the what your ADHD features are and why they react in a negative way. Once you've gotten a grip in this area, you are able to reduce your exposure to circumstances that may expose your problems or you can figure out ways to make your ADHD be beneficial to you. That is don't focus on symptoms that you don't possess. Utilize your strength to conquer those symptoms that you do have.

Concentrate on What You're Great Doing

Every one of us has something can be better than other people. If you don't have it, I believe you should take a look at your inner self. If you discover something, you should spend your time to become more proficient and skilled at what you do. It will help you feel more confident about yourself, and boost confidence in yourself.

If you can't come up with something you're proficient at, take a look at something you'd want to be proficient at and focus your efforts towards improving your performance.

Keep a positive outlook

That old saying is true. If you are prone to having more negative than positive ones, it has to be changed. If you're constantly thinking that the worst thing could happen You should begin contemplating 'what if the greatest thing occurs' instead. Positive thinking will boost your spirits both physically as well as emotionally. You'll also feel less stressed.

Always have a plan

Planning isn't easy for all. However, with time and practice it can become much easier. Begin by planning your day by creating a list of the things you want to accomplish in the day. This is a simple method of planning that can also serve as a framework. If you have a plan, you are usually able to accomplish more quickly .....and at a lower stress.

Challenge yourself

Every now and again you should step outside your comfortable zone to test your self to something that might normally find uncomfortable. It doesn't need to be something as drastic like sky diving (unless you're really keen to give it a go!). It could be eating at a an alternative eateries and taking a train trip to a new location and walking through the neighborhood at 2.30am early in the day, or something else. These kinds of activities help to develop you as an individual. You might not like every moment however, there might be a few you enjoy. It's always good to discover something new to do you enjoy!

Only work when you need To

Make sure you stick to your regular timetable. There will be occasions that you're required to work longer hours, however, these are only allowed if there is no other option. If you're able to, refuse. This is part of following a schedule that remains the same for as long as it is possible. If you are able to do the normal Monday-to- Friday, and then take weekends free, it makes things that isn't work-related much easier and more peaceful.

Enjoy A Night Out

It's nice to go out for a night with family or friends. Going to the cinema to watch some cheesy films with a friend is a wonderful option to unwind and have a good time for a short time.

Participate in a weekly class

This could be a nighttime course to discover something new or even a gym program to keep healthy, a book group or book club, etc. It is helpful to find a reason to get out of your house every week to do something productive. It's also a good method of meeting new people.

Keep a Journal

Keep a notebook or a diary and record your thoughts and experiences each day. This allows you to look at the actions you take from an entirely different point of view. It can also assist you determine if troubling patterns are beginning to appear.

Write in it each throughout the day. It'll only take you 10 minutes. You don't need to worry about grammar or spelling as it's only to keep your records.

Meditation

Although I'm no expert on meditation , but I know it works for the majority of people. There are many basic forms of meditation, and they go beyond the boundaries in this guide. However, there's lots of information available online to help you get to get started.

Take the initiative to step away from the Computer

Internet and computers are excellent for people with ADHD. Many of us who are looking at computers screens after midnight. Because the computer is something which stimulates our brains and can be a trigger for the brain, it's not a good to use the computer for more than 2 minutes before getting to bed.So make it a habit of shutting off your device at the least 2 hours prior to when you are scheduled to go to bed. This will enable your brain to start an unnatural process of slowing down and provide you with a more restful night's sleeping.

Chapter 15: Practical Everyday Strategies

If you suffer from ADHD It can be difficult to focus for a longer durations of time. It's easy to become distracted and lose your focus. There are a lot of little things you can do to assist yourself in daily life. These do not require any effort at all, nor from those who are diagnosed as well as from the family members. Here , I'll describe 10 simple strategies that you can use throughout your day life:

Utilize a quarter or half hour every morning to plan your day. In your calendar, write down tasks. It is beneficial using electronic calendars. Google calendar is an excellent alternative. The benefit of using e-calendars is that they are always accessible, anytime, anyplace. You can connect the calendar to your companion. This can prevent the double booking. Set an alarm for the date, so that you don't forget about it.

Split tasks into smaller pieces and record them in the form of a list. Be sure to write the tasks in detail. For instance, not write: "Cleaning". It is better to make an outline that looks like this:

A) "Wipe off the panel of the kitchen"

b) "Vacuum kitchen floor"

C) "Wash your kitchen's floor"

(d) "Wipe the floors in the bathroom"

(e.g.) "Polish on the mirror of the bathroom"

f) ... etc.

Include small, fun activities between you can alternate chores and enjoyment. So, it's more diverse, not just one long clean-up session. Add these lists to the computer so that they can be printed out and reused.

Schedule time every day in your calendar for routine activities. For instance, write: "Cooking from pm. 17:00-18:00"; "Put children to bed at 19:30-20.00:" Respect your personal schedule so that you don't accept an event when there's already a plan in the calendar.

Incorporate the chores that are fixed to be completed for each day. For instance, it could be beneficial to set a specific day to wash clothes. It is important to note it in your calendar, and possibly set an alarm.

Make shopping lists prior to going for a shopping trip. It is advantageous to input this information into your computer. Make sure to write the things that have been fixed on the top of the list, including dairy and bread. Create blank lines and fill in the rest with your own hand. So, you'll be able to make the same list each when you shop.

Draw an outline of the layout of your store. Draw shelves, aisles and aisles. create a list of actions as an "treasure maps". Note where you can locate the things you'll have to purchase. This way, you will be able to be sure to purchase the items you require and not get distracted.

Always keep a recording device with you or notepad. This way, you can take notes or record your thoughts and ideas on the fly. If you do this, you'll have peace of mind that you can carry on whatever you are doing. Then, later, at a different time, return on your thoughts and notes. This is a huge aid in times when thoughts are overwhelming your thoughts. Once you've written it down, it's clear of your mind and kept in a secure place and that in turn brings peace.

Create a space that is permanent for your possessions. For example, you should always put your keys on the rack right in front of the door. Start it immediately when you enter the door. It can be difficult at first to make changes to old habits. Therefore, it might be beneficial to keep notes in a place that is easy to access. Place them on eye level or perhaps with a photograph that demonstrates what you have to keep in mind in this particular instance. Once you've practiced the technique several times, it becomes an everyday routine. In time, it will become so familiar that you don't need the thought. You will know that if you can't find your keys, it's because they're at their places.

Get the necessary aids to improve your daily routine. Consider buying dishwasher, a washing machine, or a robot vacuum cleaner. These are the things that will make your life easier.

Buy as much online as you can. You can also shop for groceries. There is no sound and no pressure. There are a lot of bargains these days, in which you purchase an entire basket full of weighted and measured ingredients that are brought to your door. The basket will usually include an entire menu plan for the week along with related recipes that can be easily managed.

Chapter 16: Very simple tips for managing money and Bills

Budgeting and managing money requires preparation, and planning, which is why for a large number of people suffering from ADHD this could be an issue. Many of the typical systems of management don't tend to help adults who suffer from ADHD due to their need for excessive time in the form of paper, time, and also a focus on information. If you design your own system that's easy and regular, you will be able to stay over your financial sources and also stop excessive spending, late fees as well as charges for late deadlines.

How to Take Control of Your Budget

A thorough assessment of your financial situation is the first step towards making budgeting more manageable. Begin by keeping a close eye on all costs regardless of how tiny, for the duration of the duration of a month. This will allow you to see the direction of your money. You may be shocked by the amount you spend on unnecessary things and impulse purchases. It is possible to take this snapshot of your budgeting habits to make a month-to-month budget that is based on your income and needs.

Find out the best way to avoid deviating from your budget. If, for instance, you are spending a lot of money at dining establishments, consider an eating-in option and think about time for grocery shopping and meals preparation.

How to Set Up A Simple Money managing and bill paying system

Set up a simple and organized system to help you save receipts, papers and keep track of your expenses. If you're an adult suffering from ADHD the chance to manage your banking using a computer is a gift that keeps giving. Organising your cash online means lesser paperwork, no unpleasant handwriting, and even there are no slips that get lost.

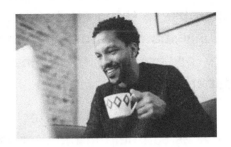

Make the switch towards online bank. Online banking could change the difficult process of managing your spending into a thing of past. Your online account will allow the entire amount of deposits and settlements, allowing you to track your balance immediately, up all the way to the penny, each day. You can also create automated payments for your normal monthly costs and then be able to make irregular or periodic ones. The most important thing is there are no envelopes lost or late fees.

Create bill payment reminders. If you prefer not to schedule automatic payments but you still can help make the process of paying much more simple by using electronic recommendations. You might be able to setup electronic mail or text suggestions through electronic banking, or program them into your calendar application.

Utilize the power of the latest technology. Free services can help in monitoring your finances and accounts. They generally take some time to setup, but when you connect to your accounts, they immediately update. They could make your financial life easier.

How to put an end to Impulse Shopping

The urge to buy caused by ADHD and buying also is a dangerous combination. It could put you in financial trouble and make you feel guilty and embarrassment. You can avoid impulsive purchases by using a few carefully planned strategies.

Cash-only shoppingLeave your checkbook at home and credit cards at your home.Cut off the equivalent of one credit card. While shopping, create your list of what you want and stick to the list.

Utilize an online calculator to keep track of the running total for purchases (tip that one is available on your mobile phone). :-).

Avoid places where you're likely to spend excessively, discard brochures when they are delivered as well as block the emails of merchants.

Tips to stay focused and efficient at work

ADHD can create unique problems at work. Some of the things that you'll find most challenging-organizing, completing tasks, staying still and paying attention in silenceThese are the things you're typically asked to complete throughout the day.

The balancing act of ADHD and a demanding job is not an simple task, however by making adjustments to your oce setting, you will be able to capitalize on your strengths while reducing the negative effects on you ADHD symptoms.

How to Stay Organized at Work

Organise your office, cubicle or workdesk. Take taking one step at a time. Utilize the following methods to keep your workspace tidy and organised:

Schedule time each day to organization.Mess is always distracting , so you should set aside 5-10 minutes every day to clean your desk and organize your papers. Look for saving points on your desk or within bins so that they don't clog your workspace with unnecessary distractions

Utilize lists and colors. Color-coding is extremely beneficial for people suffering from ADHD. Handle the issue of forgetfulness by writing down everything down.

Prioritize. The most important tasks should be rst-listed on your business order to ensure you remember to complete them before less important tasks. Make a schedule for each tiny item even if they're self-imposed.

Stop distractions

When you're faced with focus issues the place you work and what's surrounding you could dramatically determine how much you have the capacity to accomplish. Let your colleagues be aware of the need to focus and work hard. You can also try following strategies to minimize interruptions

What you do at work is crucial. If you don't have your own personal o it, you might be able to move your job to a vacant office or boardroom. If you are in an auditorium or seminar, consider sitting near the speaker and away from those who talk in the course of the discussion. Reduce the noise from outside. Your desk should be facing toward an obstruction on the wall. Also, make sure your office is clear of any clutter. To stop interruptions, place up an "Do not disturb" sign. If you are able, let your voicemail listen to your calls and return them in the future, then switch to email and social media during certain hours throughout the day. Or use your Internet completely. If you find that noise is distracting think about noise-canceling headphones or audio equipment.

Consider storing big ideas to come back the future. The amazing principles or random thoughts popping into your mind and causing you to lose focus? Note these down either on paper your smartphone to be saved for later to think about. Certain people who suffer from ADHD tend to schedule time at the end the day to review all the notes they've actually written.

How to Span your Attention span

If you're a mature adult with ADHD it is possible to focusbut you might have a difficult to keep that focus even when the subject isn't one you find particularly engaging. Talks or conferences that are monotonous are challenging for anyone, but for people who suffer from ADHD they can be an unusual challenge. In the same way, adhering to a variety of guidelines can be a challenging for people suffering from ADHD. Utilize these suggestions to increase your concentration and your ability to adhere to rules:

Make it written. If you're participating in an event or workshop, lecture, or other event that requires the attention of a specialist, request an advanced copy of relevant materials for example, a meeting agenda or summary of the lecture. When you attend the event, make use of notes in writing to guide your listening and note-taking. Making notes while you listen will help you to remain focused on the speaker's message.

Echo directions. When someone gives verbal instructions, read the instructions loudly to make sure you've got it right. Moving around. To avoid a feeling of unease and being distracted, get up and move at the proper times in the most optimal locations. If you're not causing trouble for others, consider pressing a stress ball during an event, for instance. Walking or even jumping up and down during a break in the meeting will help you focus later.

Simple Tips to Manage Stress and Enhancing Mood

Because of the impulsivity and lack of discipline that commonly occur with ADHD and ADD, you could be faced with unpredictability in your rest schedule and a sloppy diet or the effects of unproductive exerciseissues that could cause stress or moodiness, as well as feeling overwhelmed. The most effective approach to break this pattern is to be in charge of your daily habits as well as create healthy and balanced routines.

A healthy diet, plenty of rest and exercising regularly can help you remain at peace, reduce mood swings, as well as combat any signs of anxiety and clinical depression. Healthy habits can also lower ADHD symptoms like inattention, excessive activity, and distraction as well as make your life more comfortable.

Doing exercise and spending time outdoors Could help ADHD

It is a positive and effective method to reduce hyperactivity and inattention caused by ADHD. Exercise can ease tension, boost your mood, and relax your mind and help to reduce the excessive energy and anger which can create a barrier to collaboration and make it difficult to feel steady.

It is important to exercise regularly. Choose something fun and vigorous which you are able to stick with in the form of a team sport exercise routine or working out with a partner.

Increase stress relief by exercising outdoors--individuals with ADHD commonly take advantage of sunlight as well as Eco-friendly surroundings.

Find a relaxing workout such as mindful walking, yoga exercises or tai chi. In addition to calming anxiety, they can help you learn to more effectively manage your attention and your impulses.

Make sure you get enough sleep

Sleep deprivation can exacerbate the symptoms and signs of adult ADHD and reduce your ability to manage anxiety and stress as well as maintain focus during the daytime. Simple adjustments to your daytime routines can go a long way to ensuring a good night's sleep.

Avoidca einelateintheday.

Perform vigorous exercise regularly but not within an hour of going to bed.Create an organized and calm "bedtime" routine that includes taking a hot shower , or bath before going to going to bed.

Follow a regular sleep-wake schedule, even on weekends.

Consume a balanced diet

Although unhealthy eating habits are not the cause of ADHD but a poor diet can exacerbate signs. If you make simple modifications on what you eat, and what you eat you could see significant reductions in distraction and attention de cit disorder and anxiety and stress levels.

Eattinymealsthroughoutday.

Beware of sugar and convenience foods in the extent feasible.Ensure you have protein of a healthy source throughout your meal.Aim at several servings of whole grains with ber-rich content daily.

Learn to use mindfulness in helping those with ADHD

Alongside decreasing stress, regular meditation can also help you in standing against distractions, reduce the impulsivity of your mind, improve your focus and provide more control over your feelings. Given that signs of hyperactivity can make meditation difficult for people who suffer from ADHD Beginning slowly could help. Do a few minutes of meditation and gradually increase your re ection duration when you are more at ease with the method and are more adept at retaining concentration. The key is to apply these methods of mindfulness throughout your daily routine to keep you on track. You can try out absolutely free or inexpensive mobile apps and online guided meditations.

Conclusion

I hope that this book is helpful in helping you consider your illness in a new light and also determine the best ways to improve your condition. This isn't a simple process however, with enough perseverance and the support of your family and friends This is something that is feasible. Make sure to keep your head high through the whole process.

It is the next stage to implement the lessons you've learned, take it into action, and make changes to improve your life.

Thanks and best of luck!

CPSIA information can be obtained
at www.ICGtesting.com
Printed in the USA
LVHW081300290323
742838LV00003B/508

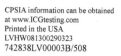

9 781774 852927